DO YOU KNOW ...

◇ Which test for prostate cancer is NOT recommended?

◇ What telephone numbers you should call *for immediate action* in the days following the diagnosis?

◇ The checklist that helps determine if the doctor is right for the patient?

◇ What specifically to say to a child about the patient's illness

◇ The coping strategies that relieve stress and manage emotions—in *both* caregiver and patient?

◇ Why a daily journal is an essential tool in healing especially for men?

◇ Why bring a tape recorder along during doctor visits?

◇ How to maximize your role as a team member for the best possible treatment decisions?

◇ How to handle the nitty-gritty realities of sex and intimacy?

◇ Which tips help alleviate incontinence—and the exercise regimen that works?

◇ How you, the caregiver, can guard ag̶a̶i̶ and maintain your peace of mind dur̶ first year?

Find out in this invaluable guide ...

Men, Women, and Prostate Cancer:
A Medical and Psychological Guide for Women and the Men They Love

Men, Women, and Prostate Cancer

A Medical and Psychological Guide
for Women and the Men They Love

BARBARA RUBIN WAINRIB, Ed.D.

SANDRA HABER, Ph.D.

WITH JACK MAGUIRE

Foreword by Michael Droller, M.D.,
Mount Sinai Medical Center, New York

New Harbinger Publications, Inc.

Publisher's Note

This publication is designed to provide accurate and authoritative information in regard to the subject matter covered. It is sold with the understanding that the publisher is not engaged in rendering psychological, financial, legal, or other professional services. If expert assistance or counseling is needed, the services of a competent professional should be sought.

Distributed in the U.S.A. by Publishers Group West; in Canada by Raincoast Books; in Great Britain by Airlift Book Company, Ltd.; in South Africa by Real Books, Ltd.; in Australia by Boobook; and in New Zealand by Tandem Press.

The first edition of this book was published by Dell Publishing in 1996 under the title *Prostate Cancer: A Guide for Women and the Men They Love.*

Cover design © 2000 by Lightbourne Images
Cover photo by George Shelly
Text design by Tracy Marie Powell

Library of Congress Catalog Card Number: 99-75278
ISBN 1-57224-182-9 Paperback

New Harbinger Publications' Web site address: www.newharbinger.com

02   01   00

10   9   8   7   6   5   4   3   2   1

First printing

This book in its revised edition is dedicated ...

To the Us Too! prostate cancer organization for self-help advocacy efforts through education and communication.

To the Us Too! board of directors who generously permitted the interviews upon which this book was based.

To the Us Too! partners who valiantly share in their partner's battles with prostate cancer and generously shared their stories with us.

Men and women live in a delicate ecology. Illness is only one factor that can threaten this balance: drastic change in the work roles of one member, particularly the traditionally nurturant caretaker, can do the same. In acknowledgment of their acceptance, encouragement, and emotional support through the months and years this project invaded our private family time, we want to dedicate this book to our husbands, Charles Kurt Wainrib and Ronald Dannenberg.

Foreword

by Michael Droller, M.D.

This year, 40,000 American men will die of prostate cancer, and 175,000 new cases will be diagnosed. The explosive increase in such figures over the past twenty years has catapulted prostate cancer to prominence as one of the major U.S. health problems today.

As screening becomes more commonplace, the number of diagnoses is expected to rise even more dramatically during the foreseeable future. The greater health consciousness of Americans in general, the growing publicity generated by well-known men with prostate cancer, and the ever more intense focus placed on the "prostate cancer epidemic" by the media are drawing widening attention not only to the illness itself, but also to the storms of controversy that have arisen regarding its diagnosis, its characterization, and its treatment.

Is the recent increase in casualties due to a rise in specific health-threatening factors, or does it simply represent the enhanced ability of doctors to diagnose the condition at an earlier stage in its development, thanks to tests that were previously unavailable? Has the disease somehow become more devastating than it was in years gone by, or are men just living longer and therefore running a greater risk of eventually having it?

It is clear that cancer can kill. At the same time, there are many men diagnosed with prostate cancer who never actually suffer from it. This latter fact, however, is small assurance for those who hear the words: "You have prostate cancer."

This book addresses many of the questions that a man and his loved ones face when they learn that he has prostate cancer. Although medical science does not have all the answers, and many of the issues involving prostate cancer remain controversial, a patient and his family must seek to be informed as much as possible about what is known and what is not known. Only then can they be fully equipped to make effective decisions—perhaps the most important ones they will ever have to make.

The authors of this book have taken particular pains to explore every aspect of the concerns that patients and their loved ones will have when confronted with the diagnosis of prostate cancer. These concerns are discussed in an unbiased, comprehensive, and understandable manner. The discussions are based on the most current knowledge available, and are presented from the standpoint of "What do the patient and his loved ones need to know?"

The success of any interaction between patient and physician requires sound knowledge, understandable knowledge, and the transmission of both with compassion, sensitivity, and support. These same requirements underlie interactions that develop between a person confronted with a potentially life-threatening illness and those on whom he or she relies in dealing with it. This book offers valuable help in meeting all of these requirements. Any patient with prostate cancer, and anyone confronted with this problem in somebody they love, will derive great comfort in reading and rereading this book to seek answers for the many questions that they must be prepared to face.

Contents

Acknowledgments

(for the second edition)

We want to thank the caring, patient folks at New Harbinger: Matthew McKay and Patrick Fanning for showing their interest in our work over the years, and especially Kristin Beck for her patience, understanding, and constant support. Along with them are the whole New Harbinger team who were considerate—and human—throughout the process

(from first edition)

One of our long-standing beliefs has been in what we call the Phoenix Phenomenon, which, simply stated, says that sometimes a crisis situation can help mobilize untapped resources and allow one to redirect energies toward new goals. This book is a Phoenix product.

Our own involvement on this journey is described in the body of the book, but here we need only say that what started as a family crisis redirected our energies to what we hope is a helpful new product. We have both been working as psychologists in private practice as well as teaching at universities (B.W. at McGill in Montreal, S.H. at Adelphi in New York), publishing professional papers and books for many years. However, the events of a recent autumn laid the groundwork for this, our first mass-market book.

Had we not been allowed to share in the experiences of two couples very dear to us, this project would not have existed. And so we must first and foremost offer our gratitude to Victor Afriat and Jeannine Wainrib for allowing us to accompany them on each step of their journey through the sometimes frightening and often frustrating experience of Victor's battle with prostate cancer. As our work progressed, Victor and Jeannine were joined by many other couples from all over North America with whom we spent hundreds of hours of interview time. These were people who came forward to talk to us about their prostate cancer experience as both patients and spouses. We are deeply grateful to all of them. In particular we want to thank the board of directors of Us Too, who so generously gave of their time and energy to help nurture the seedling project. Members, along with their partners, gave us a full understanding of both the male and the female experience of this illness.

Resource people for this book, like the illness itself, were widespread. Talking to many of these people reinforced our belief in the essential goodness and generosity of human beings.

In Montreal we are grateful to Dr. Eva Libman and Dr. Zeev Rosberger, both psychologists at the Jewish General Hospital, for their time, information, and direction. We want to thank Isabelle Gregoire, R.N., of the prostate cancer support group and the Hope and Cope group, also at the Jewish General Hospital, and Rhona Small, M.S.W., and the Cancer Hot Line for their cooperation as well. I am also grateful to Dean Rachelle Keyserlingk of McGill University, who encouraged me to launch a graduate course in psychooncology as this work progressed.

In Los Angeles, we are deeply grateful to Pat Turcillo of the UCLA prostate cancer program. Pat's wonderful spirit of caring and understanding and her willingness to talk to us at great length whenever needed were exceptional. Her referral of many of her group members to us for interviews was most helpful as well. We are also grateful to her for inviting us to her group to present our communication workshop for prostate couples. Also in Los Angeles, our thanks go to Arie Belledegrun, M.D., F.A.C.S., professor of urology at UCLA.

And in New York our deep gratitude goes to Carolyn Messner, C.S.W., director of New York Cancer Care, as well as to Josephine Di Verniere, C.S.W., director, and Carol Becker, support group leader, both of the Cancer Institute of Brooklyn at Maimonides Hospital. At Memorial Sloan-Kettering Cancer Center we wish to thank Dr. Jimmie Holland and Dr. Bill Breitbart of the Network project as well as Les Gallo-Silver, C.S.W., of the prostate support group. On the technical end, Richie Gutwirth spent many hours perfecting the music portion of our relaxation tape.

Also in New York are three people essential to this project. First and foremost is Faith Hamlin, our agent, cheerleader, nurturer, and true believer, who shepherded and sheltered us in the world of trade publishing. She introduced us to Jack Maguire, who helped translate our ideas and understanding of human relationships into practical, readable suggestions. Faith was also a conduit to Dr. Michael Droller, professor and chairman of the Department of Urology of the Mount Sinai Medical Center, who provided the essential medical expertise. And our most crucial New York connection, Steve Ross, our editor at Dell, and Mollie Doyle, his delightful, dependable assistant.

The serendipity yield has been great in this project as well. Had Dr. Dorothy Cantor, current president of the American Psychological Association, not met Barbara in 1988 and welcomed her in to the Gender Issues Committee, she and Sandy might never have met. And had Dr. Lauren Ayres not made her passionate speech about women and breast cancer at a divisional midwinter meeting, their collaboration on *Breast Cancer: A Psychological Treatment Manual* might never have occurred. And had Dr. Richard Mikesell, then president of the Division of Independent Practice, not supported Sandy in spearheading the writing of the *Manual*, the present book might never have been conceived.

Early on in this project prominent individuals like Senator Bob Dole and Michael Milken had the courage to publicize their own struggles with prostate cancer, which set the tone for a public awareness of the prevalence of this illness.

Connections and partnerships came in all forms, and we wish to thank Dr. Pat DeLeon for his wisdom and mentoring within the political process. As a psychologist and assistant to Senator Daniel Inouye, he has underscored the contribution of psychology in medical illness and other areas to an audience as influential as the United States Congress.

In addition, we want to thank the many members of the Division of Independent Practice of the American Psychological Association who are not only colleagues but friends and a multi-faceted support system for both of us. Too numerous to mention individually, their lives are, nonetheless, inextricably interwoven with our own. Our many personal friends and relatives outside of APA helped us stay the course, even in the hardest times.

Last but never least is our appreciation of the backup of our families. Sandy is fortunate that her parents, Marilyn and Irwin, provide her with an admirable model of aging. Our sons, both Andrews (Haber and Wainrib), and our daughters, Samantha Dannenberg and Jeannine Wainrib, as well as Jeannine's husband, Victor Afriat, and my granddaughter, Rachel Wainrib Friendly, help us create a "safe place" for our existence in this busy world. We value their input, love, caring, and generational balance. Our network of siblings and siblings-in-law is always there for us. Our husbands, Charles K. Wainrib and Ronald Dannenberg, to whom this book is dedicated, know that it is far more than their exper-tise in technology and the "Information Highway" for which we applaud them. And, in keeping with our multifaceted concept of "healing partnerships," we also want to acknowledge the ever-present warmth, adoration, and spiritual support of Champ and Mokie.

October 1995   Barbara Rubin Wainrib, Ed.D.,
                Clinical Psychologist
                Associate Professor, McGill University
                Private Practice, Montreal

                Sandra Haber, Ph.D.,
                Psychologist
                Associate Clinical Professor, Derner Institute,
                Adelphi University
                Private Practice, New York City

1

The Healing
Partnership

⬥ Prostate cancer's special impact on men

⬥ The critical role of the caregiver

⬥ The effect of prostate cancer on relationships

⬥ Healing versus curing

Men don't want to talk about it. They may think it can't happen to them. They may think it only happens to old men who are dying anyway. Or they may think it invariably leads to impotence and incontinence—unspeakable propositions.

All of these notions are wrong. According to the American Cancer Society (ACS), more than 140,000 new cases of prostate cancer are diagnosed in the United States each year, and one in ten men in the United States develops cancer in the semen-producing prostate gland, almost the same incidence as breast cancer among women; and 20 percent of these men are, according to the U.S. Census Bureau middle-aged (forty to sixty-five years old). In 1994, it was second only to lung cancer as the leading cancer killer among American men.

Contrary to popular opinion, if prostate cancer is caught early and treated effectively, it doesn't have to mean death, impotence, or incontinence. But male denial works against early detection and effective treatment. Forty-three percent of doctors surveyed by the American Medical Association in 1992 claimed that men with prostate cancer go untreated merely because they don't want to talk about it with their doctors. An astounding 85 percent of doctors surveyed said that even men who *do* talk about prostate cancer are not prepared to cope with it well— pragmatically or psychologically.

What happens when a middle-aged man, facing all sorts of new concerns about his virility, suddenly discovers that he has prostate cancer? How does he go about confronting a disease that attacks the source of his manhood, and threatens to destroy his bladder control, his sexual capabilities, his very life? Where does he turn for help?

In the overwhelming majority of cases, men in this situation turn to the women in their lives. Indeed, men facing *any* illness generally depend upon women to research that illness, supervise day-to-day care, provide emotional relief, and, inevitably, do most of the talking to family, friends, and health-care professionals. This is true even when the sickness is relatively minor. A popular television commercial glorifies "Dr. Mom," whose young children and adult husband are equally dependent upon her—physically and emotionally—to deal with their common colds. Another familiar commercial depicts a rugged-looking fly fisherman stifling his reaction to pain in his hands, while the voice-over tells us that when he gets arthritis, his wife gives him a pain reliever. Sadly, we understand the twisted logic involved: It wouldn't fit the fly fisherman's macho image if he were to get the pain reliever for himself!

In keeping with this reality, this book is primarily addressed to the women who care for men during this illness. Even though this book also offers valuable, comprehensive information and guidance for male readers—caregivers as well as patients—it makes a special effort to address the unique concerns of the wives, mothers, daughters, granddaughters, sisters, daughters-in-law, sisters-in-law, nieces, aunts, and/or female life-companions, lovers, or friends in a stricken man's life who work alone or, more commonly, in a supportive female network to tend to the man's physical, practical, and psychological needs. It squarely acknowledges what all the research on the subject confirms: In our society, it is usually women who wind up managing most healthcare issues relating to men's illnesses, resulting in a healing partnership that's inextricably involved with gender-related issues as well.

A case in point is that of U.S. Senate Majority Leader Bob Dole, who, after having his prostate cancer surgically removed in 1992, has campaigned so vigorously for prostate cancer awareness that he's become, in his own words, "the prostate pinup boy." In relying on the primary woman in his life to deal with his cancer crisis, Dole was luckier than most men in one respect: He's married to the then head of the American Red Cross. So when he turned to his wife, Elizabeth Dole, for help, something he admitted to a *People* magazine reporter that he does "instinctively" anytime he's feeling "stunned, pressured, or plain old sick," she could immediately call personal contacts in top medical centers around the country for advice.

Not all wives have such connections. As Dole has come to realize through his frequent talks in public forums, prostate cancer is an illness that "strikes couples and families, not simply individuals," and "people are just hungry for information."

In effect, Dole did for prostate cancer what former First Lady Betty Ford did almost two decades ago for breast cancer: brought it to the forefront of national attention and instilled among American men *and* women a desire for more and better materials on what to do about it. In the wake of Dole, other well-known men have also stepped forward to confirm the key role played by the women in their lives in dealing with their illness, and to plead for better patient-caregiver education. Among these men have been Len Dawson, Hall of Fame quarterback and television sportscaster, who admits that he would not even have had the checkup that discovered his cancer except for his wife's insistence; Jerry Lewis, comedian; Don Ameche, actor; Linus Pauling, scientist and two-time Nobel-prize winner; Frank Zappa, rock musician; Joseph Papp, theatrical producer; Robert Penn Warren, writer and the nation's first poet laureate; Roone Arledge, president of ABC news; John Paul Stevens, U.S. Supreme Court Justice; Jim Berry, nationally syndicated cartoonist; and Steven Ross, chairman of Time Warner.

Over the past few years, these prominent spokespeople have contributed to a groundswell of interest in prostate cancer, while at the same time revolutionary breakthroughs in detection and treatment have occurred. Successive refinements in measuring the level of prostate specific antigen (PSA) in a man's bloodstream have led to a relatively simple, inexpensive, and comfortable means of testing for the possible presence of prostate cancer (as discussed in chapter 3 of this book). And a sophisticated "nerve-sparing" surgical technique can now sharply reduce the risk of impotence associated with cancerous prostate gland removal (as discussed in chapters 4, 6, and 8).

Unfortunately, each of these highly significant medical advances has generated its own maelstrom of controversy, which only further perplexes today's patients and their caregivers. Because prostate cancer is typically very slow to grow, a man who has a small tumor may live a long, healthy life and die of some other natural cause (including advanced age) long before the cancer can become a problem. Thus, early detection—now made more possible by PSA testing—often raises agonizing questions: Should an early-Stage C/T3 or T4 cancer be treated aggressively, in which case the patient may run an unnecessary risk of impotence and incontinence, or should the patient simply put off treatment, waiting to see what develops over time, in which case he may wind up risking his life?

As for the nerve-sparing surgical technique, many conservative medical experts warn that its actual success rate has not been accurately determined. In the meantime, they say, exaggerated claims about its effectiveness are influencing many patients and their caregivers to look, more favorably than they should, upon surgery as a treatment option.

Amid all the welcome new attention to prostate cancer and the promising, if controversial, new medical developments in its detection and treatment, patients and their female caregivers are still challenged as much as ever by certain basic problems. It is these matters, often allowed to lurk in the darkness, that this book is dedicated to illuminating. Such problems include the following:

> *It remains extremely difficult to predict how a given case of prostate cancer will develop and to determine how best to treat it, which makes each case unique.*

The prostate gland itself is one of the least understood parts of the male anatomy. Its small size and its deeply embedded position within the body complicate research efforts, and scientists still have many questions about its biological purpose and function, its puzzling tendency to grow increasingly larger as a man ages, and the reasons why the course of prostate cancer can vary so much from individual to individual. Adding to the gland's mystery is the fact that men down through the ages have been so reluctant to talk about trouble "down there," out of fear, embarrassment, or false bravado.

As a result of all this ignorance and uncertainty, there are extremely few "general truths" about prostate cancer. Each individual case must be considered unique; and, because different, equally qualified doctors often disagree strongly on how to treat the same case, patients and their caregivers often need to play a greater-than usual role in determining for themselves how they want to handle illness-related matters. Even more so than with other serious diseases, specific treatment decisions about prostate cancer must take into account the individual patient's overall physical condition, emotional well-being, psychological resources, living situation, and lifestyle preferences.

> *From the man's perspective, the stress associated with prostate cancer diagnosis and treatment can easily aggravate stress relating to other psychological issues involving his manhood and aging.*

One of the cruelest ironies about prostate cancer is that it usually strikes men at that time in their life when they're most concerned about their virility: between the ages of fifty and sixty-five. This concern—part conscious and part subconscious—is much more multidimensional than a simple "midlife crisis" about getting older, being "outdone" by younger men, and possibly not having realized certain lifelong dreams. It's a complex reaction to a number of symptoms that may well be associated with a natural drop in male hormone levels. Scientists are now in the process of verifying that most men during this age period go through a kind of hitherto unacknowledged, ignored, or denied "male menopause," a condition that has been dubbed "viropause" in the medical literature.

Although viropause is certainly milder in its observable effects than menopause, it can be similarly upsetting to the individual. Physically, men going through viropause experience greater and more frequent fatigue; a decline in muscle mass, tone, and strength; and a waning of their "youth-related" attractiveness. Emotionally, they find themselves increasingly beset by fear, depression, and confusion. But one of the most disturbing developments of all is inseparably physical *and* emotional in nature: a decline in sexual desire and potency.

To varying degrees, most men in this age bracket find themselves having unprecedented or much more frequent problems getting or sustaining an erection—a situation that medical investigators over the past decade have often been able to link to declining hormone levels. Comedian George Burns was able to laugh about this problem when it began happening to him: "Everything that goes up must come down," he joked, "but there comes a time when not everything that's down can come up." Most men who develop the problem, however, are not so even tempered in their response. They can't help worrying to some extent about losing their manhood altogether—perhaps sooner rather than later. When they're diagnosed with prostate cancer, such fears can compound exponentially.

Then there's the issue of retirement. Many men who are diagnosed with prostate cancer are in the process of ending a lifetime of productive work: either they're planning to retire in the near future, or they've just recently retired and are still adjusting to their new, "nonproductive" status. Both situations leave a man vulnerable to occasional feelings of insecurity, worthlessness, and despair about the future. These feelings, too, can become much more frequent and powerful if the man also has to worry about the fact that he has prostate cancer.

From a couple's perspective, the stress associated with living through the prostate cancer experience can put an enormous burden on their relationship.

Couples and, indeed, whole families can suffer in all sorts of unexpected ways from an individual's serious illness. Jane E. Brody, reporter on medical subjects for *The New York Times,* describes how far reaching the effects can be:

When someone in the family develops a chronic, disabling, incurable, or life-threatening disorder, everyone in the family is likely to get "sick" as well. Aspirations and plans of the spouse and children, as well as the affected person, must often be readjusted, and roles within the family structure must be redefined. Communication patterns change, and not always for the better, and the resulting emotional, physical, financial stresses can strain even the most stable relationships.

In terms of an intimate relationship, the man's prostate cancer can have an especially devastating impact, presenting a constant, insidious threat to the couple's ability to make love, enjoy physical closeness, and rely on the life-supporting roles that they've established for themselves.

Men and women live together in a very delicate ecology of cooperation and opposition. When a crisis hits, their coping skills are overloaded and their usual mechanisms of relating to each other break down. Never is good communication more essential between them, and never is it more difficult to maintain. Difficulties in transmitting and receiving information that may have been unrecognized or overlooked in easier times now loom large and menacing.

Many male-female communication problems are not simply interpersonal in nature but have to do with socialized gender distinctions. The way men are raised and come to envision life is typically different from the way women are raised and come to envision life; as a result, differing, gender-related modes of communication emerge.

For example, Dr. Jean Baker Miller, a prominent psychiatrist and authority on the subject, has found that when a woman talks with another woman, each is predisposed to respond to the other with empathy and to relate to the other person as someone who shares a "woman's agenda." This serves to give the two women a sense of connectedness—a psychological state that women in general have been culturally conditioned to seek in order to avoid social isolation. Two men, by contrast, are more likely to talk to each other in a back-and-forth "point-counterpoint" manner. This gives each man a sense of individual competence and self-sufficiency—a psychological state that men in general have been culturally conditioned to seek in order to avoid feeling incompetent.

When a man and woman get together to talk, these differences can easily trigger problems that baffle both genders. For example, when a woman tells a man something that she considers important, it's very possible that he won't respond with the degree of empathy that she expects. Therefore, she may get angry and accuse him of not understanding her. In fact, the man's failure to express empathy may not mean that he doesn't think what she said was important, or that he doesn't understand her. It may be just his gender-related way of responding—or even of offering stoic "down-to-earth" help. If so, he may react to her anger with indignation about being falsely accused.

In the popular 1992 book *Men Are from Mars, Women Are from Venus*, Dr. John Gray discusses another common theory about the difference between male and female communication: namely, that men are less inclined to talk at all, especially during a crisis. Due to the different ways that each gender is culturally conditioned, a woman may want to talk things out as soon as a crisis hits (perhaps due to her urgent need for connectedness), while a man may first want to "go into his cave" to think things out (perhaps due to his urgent need to believe he can solve matters all by himself).

While theories vary about precisely how and why men and women have communication problems, one point is indisputable:

Men and women *do* experience life—and express that experience—in a different manner. Thus, men and their female partners going through any kind of crisis, particularly one as serious and potentially devastating as the man's prostate cancer, must take special care to understand, respect, and cope with this difference. With lots of hard work and a little luck, this special care may ultimately render the relationship even stronger than it was before the crisis struck.

Because the ultimate physical consequences of prostate cancer can be so difficult to predict or control, and because the possible emotional effects of the illness can be so devastating, it's important to place at least as much value on healing the person as curing the disease.

The process of curing prostate cancer involves ridding the body of every trace of that cancer, so that it ceases to pose a threat. It's strictly a physical procedure. It doesn't take into account the patient's emotional life, his psychological integrity, his interpersonal relationships, and/or the quality of his day-to-day existence. Whether or not there's been a cure (something that can be very difficult to effect or determine in *any* case of cancer), the odds are high that these other factors in the patient's life will also be disturbed by the illness, and in need of their own more comprehensive and creative care.

How I Became Involved
by Dr. Barbara

A few years ago, I got a telephone message from one of my best friends, who I will call Ruth, asking me to find some time to have coffee with her as soon as I could. Although Ruth is one of the most upbeat persons I know, her voice on the phone sounded teary and urgent. We connected a few nights later, and as soon as I got into her car, I said, "I know your mother just died and you're upset about that, but your message sounded as if there's something more."

"Well," said Ruth, "for one thing, Harold [her husband] has cancer!" I was shocked and horrified. A month earlier, Ruth and Harold had held a wonderful party celebrating Harold's sixtieth birthday. All of us who loved him knew that for much of his life he had lived under the pall of his father's early death at fifty-nine. But he had finally reached sixty, and, what's more, he'd received a major promotion at the same time. Now he had cancer. How nasty could the fates be?

Ruth went on to tell me what she had learned about prostate cancer. She had studiously spent the past weekend at the library getting as much information as she could. Then she told me how her kids had rallied and organized a conference call to their dad. We talked about how suddenly and irrevocably her life had changed, just at the point where it had looked as if it was going to be better than ever. We looked at the worst-case scenario for the cancer and cried. Then we looked at the best-case scenario, which, according to what the doctors had said so far, was "three lousy months." We hugged each other and said, "Here's to three lousy months—we can at least celebrate that!"

A few weeks later I got a call from my daughter, who lives three thousand miles away. To me she sounded very upset, even though she was obviously trying to sound calm. She said that when her husband's doctor examined him for a kidney stone, he found an enlargement of his prostate and did a biopsy. The doctor now wanted to see them to discuss the results. She called again after the appointment. The doctor never actually used the word *cancer,* but told them all the tests were positive and went on to describe the tumor to them. He also gave them a copy of the lab reports. Fresh from my experience with Ruth, I knew what questions to ask her, and none of the answers were good. His surgery was scheduled for a few weeks later.

The time in between was frightening for all of us, including my twelve-year-old granddaughter, my daughter's child, who had just been through a divorce and custody battle. Long telephone conversations with my granddaughter were okay, but this was a time to hold and hug, and not even Sprint can do that! Fortunately, she had a special math teacher at school to whom she could tell anything; and on the day of the surgery, she was allowed to go to a quiet place by herself. It was during this time that I called Sandy, a good friend with whom I had worked on a breast cancer manual for the American Psychological Association (now available from Springer, New York), and we decided to do a book on prostate cancer.

How I Became Involved by Dr. Sandy

Barbara, a dear friend and one of my co-authors in writing a breast cancer manual, called me one morning. She was very upset: her son-in-law had just been diagnosed with prostate cancer. "What do you know about prostate cancer?" Barbara asked.

To my own surprise, it turned out that I really didn't know very much at all. I put the telephone on hold and asked my husband, who was in the room, "What do you know about prostate cancer?" I suppose I felt that he would know a lot more about it than I did, since it's a man's illness. He just looked back at me and shrugged his shoulders. I was shocked at his lack of knowledge! I excused my own ignorance, but why did he, a man, know so little?

Determined to help my friend, I went to the bookstore near my office that very day. It's a large bookstore with a wellstocked section on health issues. I was appalled to find just two books on prostate cancer—only one of which seemed worth buying. I bought it. Then I read the entire book that day.

Much to my chagrin, after reading that book, I was still thoroughly confused. I didn't feel that I'd learned anything that could help Barbara, something I very much wanted to do. The treatment options remained unclear, and I was especially upset about the slight attention given to emotional issues. References to impotence and incontinence were sprinkled throughout the book, but they made these issues seem rather matter-of-fact when, to me and to others with whom I spoke, they were actually quite alarming issues.

In general, the book offered no sense of how "real people" might react to prostate cancer and its side effects, physical *and* emotional, nor any concrete guidance on what those real people might do about their reactions. I thought of my husband and realized that if I were trying to be a good partner to him during his prostate cancer, this book would be utterly useless. And so I called Barbara and told her my story. I promised to go to the library to search for more answers. And I told her that our book on prostate cancer had already begun.

That's where healing comes in. In the context of prostate cancer, healing involves helping the patient come to good terms with all aspects of his life: the physical condition of his prostate gland and the rest of his body, as well as his emotions, his psychological state, his interpersonal relationships, and the quality of his day-to-day existence. His cancer may not be curable, but, with proper treatment, he can go on to heal and lead an enjoyable, productive life—maybe even one that never does become physically compromised by the cancer. If, however, he does suffer physical setbacks as a result of the cancer, he can still experience healing by learning to accept his illness for what it is, and to cultivate personal well-being however and wherever he can. Only by doing so can he—or any cancer patient—start feeling "at one" with his life after it's been so seriously threatened.

Over the past several years we conducted many in-depth interviews with different kinds of patient-caregiver partnerships involved in a wide variety of prostate cancer situations. The insights gained from these interviews, from consultations with experts in the field, and from our own professional experience as therapists form the heart and soul of this book, and will assist you in coping with many of the "hidden struggles" that can attend the illness. Among these issues are:

◊ how to deal with panic, denial, anger, or other emotions that commonly arise after the diagnosis;

◊ how to build up an effective, reliable, and nurturing network of support among your family and friends;

◊ how to work constructively with doctors and other medical personnel to develop the most effective treatment program and to respond to your specific needs and desires;

◊ how to handle both practical and emotional matters having to do with impotence, incontinence, and other adverse physical effects of the illness or its treatment.

For your convenience, this book is organized according to the progress of the illness—from cause, detection, and diagnosis (chapters 2 through 5), to treatment (chapters 6, 7, and 8), to recovery from treatment (chapter 9), to posttreatment life (chapter 10). However, regardless of where you and your partner now find yourselves along this continuum, you will both benefit greatly from reading the entire book. Many physical, emotional, psychological, and interpersonal matters that become critically important during a later phase of the illness have their origin in an earlier phase.

The more informed you are about prostate cancer as a whole, the better able you will be to manage each and every day of living with it. So little is known for sure about the illness, and so many myths circulate, that every bit of understanding you can bring to your experience of it will be enormously valuable to you, your doctor, and your loved ones.

2

Why and How Prostate Cancer Develops

- ⬥ The purpose and function of the gland
- ⬥ Common noncancerous prostate disorders: prostatitis and benign prostate hyperplasia (BPH)
- ⬥ Factors that may cause prostate cancer
- ⬥ Prostate cancer's stages of growth

Scientists and laypeople alike marvel that a gland so tiny, smaller than the average walnut, can be the cause of so much trouble for men. Regrettably, much about the prostate gland, and how prostate cancer develops, is mysterious.

In this chapter, we will try to shed some light on that mystery and, in doing so, help you come to a better understanding of what happens inside a man's body when prostate cancer strikes. It's not the easiest information to absorb mentally or emotionally, partly because it's dry and technical, and partly because so many important pieces of the puzzle are still missing, including "What does the prostate gland *really* do for a man?" "Isn't there *any* way that prostate cancer can be avoided?" and the most maddening question of all, "Why do the possible consequences of prostate cancer have to be so devastating?"

Nevertheless, hard to absorb as the information may be, it is crucial to the prostate cancer patient's peace of mind and to your peace of mind as the patient's primary caregiver. A good, basic knowledge of the biophysical environment in which the illness is taking place will help both of you to keep your bearings as you wade through all the data you'll encounter relating to diagnosis, treatment, and recovery.

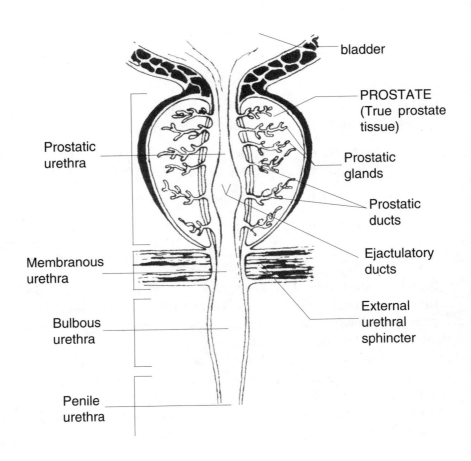

The word *prostate* itself comes from the Greek words for "stand before." Coined in the sixteenth century by the French surgeon Ambroise Paré, a pioneer in the study of the prostate, the term was meant to describe the gland's role as Paré perceived it: "gatekeeper for the bladder."

True, the prostate does surround a portion of the urethra—the tubelike structure that carries urine from the bladder to the penis. This portion of the urethra—known as the prostatic urethra—lies directly below the bladder itself and just before the external urethral sphincter, the muscle that a man can voluntarily contract to stop his flow of urine during urination. But in its normal state, the prostate gland does nothing to affect the flow of urine through the prostatic urethra—a fact that belies its gatekeeper label.

The true picture of the prostate gland's functional relationship to the bladder is much grimmer. When the gland becomes overly enlarged because of illness or advanced age (for unknown reasons, the prostate grows slowly, at varied paces, throughout a man's lifetime), it can cause erratic or chronic pinching, blocking, and backing up of the urine flowing out of the bladder. Down through the ages, this particular problem has been the most obvious signal not only of trouble in the gland but also of the gland's very existence.

Although the prostate gland may, in a diseased state, play an active role as "gatekeeper for the bladder," the role for which nature apparently intended it has to do with a man's reproductive functioning. Besides carrying urine when a man urinates, the urethra also transports semen that comes from the seminal vesicle when a man ejaculates (during which time a small, involuntarily controlled sphincter temporarily closes off the bladder). After the semen passes into the prostatic urethra, it is augmented slightly by secretions from the prostate gland. Actually, these secretions, each different in kind, are produced by numerous small, independent glands housed within the muscular and fibrous casing that we call, for convenience's sake, the prostate gland.

Just what these prostatic secretions do—individually or collectively—for the male reproductive function is not yet known. Most scientists assume that they help nourish the sperm, which

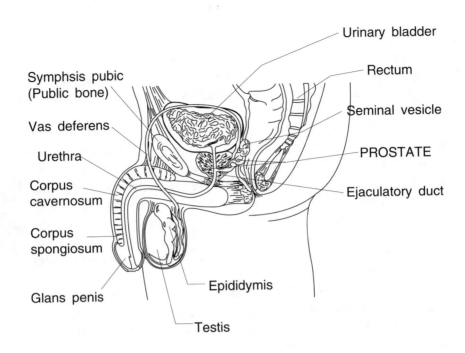

enter the semen stream later, from the testicles; but sperm can survive without these secretions, so they aren't considered to be essential for fertility.

The gland as a whole also appears to contribute to the male orgasm. Together with the muscles surrounding the urethra, the prostate gland contracts at the moment of ejaculation to produce the thrust that sends the semen down through the urethra, where it picks up sperm from the testicles before shooting out of the penis. However, men can experience an orgasm without a prostate gland (and even without an erection—a fact that many men don't realize; see chapter 4 for further discussion).

Tiny as the prostate gland may be, and small as its normal role may be in reproduction, it can still trigger problems with enormous consequences, including total and irreversible incontinence, infertility, and/or impotency. Later in this chapter, we will discuss how prostate cancer can, at times, lead to death. For now, let's look briefly at the various *noncancerous* disorders of the prostate and what relationship (if any) they have to prostate cancer.

Prostatitis

Prostatitis, literally meaning "inflammation of the prostate," is a very general term covering a number of different kinds of conditions that are not life threatening but nevertheless are potentially very painful and aggravating. The simplest form of prostatitis is a mild, noninfectious irritation known as "prostatodynia," which can often be linked to stress and is generally treated with anti-inflammatory medications or muscle relaxants. More frequently, prostatitis results from an infection caused by microorganisms that travel up the urethra from the penis. In many cases both the prostatic urethra and the prostate are infected by these microorganisms; in some cases, only the prostatic urethra is actually infected, but the condition is still considered to be prostatitis. Among the most common infectious agents are coliform bacteria and the types of bacteria that can also cause staphylococcus infections, sexually transmitted diseases, tuberculosis, and vaginal yeast infections.

A widespread complaint among men of all ages, and one of the major reasons why a man visits a doctor, infection-related prostatitis is like a "cold" in the prostate. Often it comes and goes without the man even being aware of it. A mild case may cause a vague, indefinable discomfort in the penis (the pain of most cases of prostatitis is felt in the penis, rather than the prostate itself, due to so-called "associative pain," whereby the pain signal, traveling along nerves extending from the prostate to the penis, consciously registers as coming from the penis).

Symptoms of more serious infections include the following:

◊   sharp, searing pain during urination;

◊   persistent throbbing along the underside of the penis;

◊   bloody or pus-laden discharge during urination or ejaculation;

◊   dull, continual pain across the groin or lower back; and/or

◊   an overall feeling of malaise or weakness.

Some cases of prostatitis are short term and intense (technically, "acute prostatitis"), others are long term and relatively moderate (technically, "chronic prostatitis," with the possibility of intermittent attacks of acute symptoms).

Almost all cases of infection-related prostatitis can be successfully treated with antibiotics, and sometimes bed rest. Unfortunately, many men delay treatment or avoid it altogether, preferring simply to "tough it out." To the man himself, this can seem like a reasonable course of action because the pain of even a serious infection can quickly fade to a tolerable level or disappear for fairly lengthy periods of time. The trouble is that the infection, though no longer discomforting, may remain just as extensive and vigorous, ultimately spreading to cause even greater damage and more distressing symptoms.

Experts are currently studying whether there is any connection between prostatitis and prostate cancer. To date, no evidence has emerged to indicate that men who have had prostatitis are more—or less—likely to develop prostate cancer. The two types of illness, prostatitis and prostate cancer, still appear to be entirely unrelated to each other.

However, when it comes to detection of, and recovery from, prostate cancer, there may very well be one significant difference between men who have been treated for prostatitis and men who have not. Men who feel compelled to go to a urologist because of their prostatitis, especially if they go on a recurring basis, are often tested by the urologist for other prostate disorders, including prostate cancer. The same men are also predisposed to visit a urologist whenever they have *any* urinogenital discomfort. Ironically, these circumstances alone may mean that men who undergo treatment for prostatitis and who also develop prostate cancer are more likely to have their cancer detected at an early, more treatable stage of growth than men who have never had prostatitis and therefore have never taken the time and effort to see a urologist. The bottom line is that men should have a urological checkup periodically—at least once a year after age forty—to determine if they have any prostate disorder, regardless of whether they do or do not have symptoms.

Benign Prostatic Hyperplasia (BPH)

The prostate gland naturally enlarges with age. It doesn't swell because of a tumor, but simply grows bigger from within, at the core of the prostate surrounding the prostatic urethra. According to the American Medical Association, in about 35 percent of men over fifty years old, 50 percent of men over sixty, and 65 percent of men over seventy, this enlargement starts squeezing the prostatic urethra, possibly causing discomfort, at which time the gland's growth process—still natural and benign in itself—is deemed a disorder known as "benign prostatic hyperplasia" (BPH).

In the popular imagination, BPH is often confused with prostate cancer, which is a much less common and much more serious condition featuring a malignant tumor A major cause of this confusion is the tendency of many people to refer to either condition merely as "prostate trouble," not wanting to talk more specifically about something that embarrasses them. Adding to the confusion is the fact that the symptoms of BPH are similar in kind to some of the possible symptoms of prostate cancer:

- ◊ a thinning of the urinary stream, so that it takes a much longer time to urinate;

- ◊ a need to strain to empty the bladder;

- ◊ a failure to empty the bladder completely, resulting in a more frequent need to urinate (which is especially disruptive of nighttime sleep); and/or

- ◊ the intermittent occurrence of a sudden, intense pressure to urinate that can be very difficult to resist and, when the man is in the company of other people, very embarrassing.

(More information on the symptoms, detection, and diagnosis of prostate cancer follows in the next chapter.)

Some men—either fearing that their BPH might be prostate cancer or just wanting to avoid the nuisance of medical intervention—try ignoring the difficulties of BPH as long as they can, which only makes matters worse. In addition to more severe urination problems, perhaps ultimately resulting in the man's inability to urinate at all without a catheter, the delay may result in painful complications caused by the stalled urine itself. As this urine lingers in the bladder, it can begin to stagnate, perhaps assisting the development of already present bacteria that may then go on to infect the entire urinary tract. Also, if the amount of urinary "backflow" becomes relatively large, it can exert pressure on the kidneys that may lead to irreversible kidney damage.

Doctors have recently had a limited amount of success treating BPH with drugs designed to shrink or soften prostate gland tissue. *Proscar* is the trade name of the most often used drug (developed by Merck Laboratories); alternatively, a class of drugs called alpha-blockers may be prescribed. Proscar (finasteride) is the most often used drug to "shrink" the prostate, potentially leading to a 25–40 percent decrease in size. This drug has minimal side effects. Alpha-blockers appear to "relax" the bladder outlet smooth muscle as well as the smooth muscle fibers of the prostate, allowing a freer flow of urine. A substantial number of men (20–30 percent) experience lightheadedness or fatigue with alpha-blockers. A new product known as "flomax" may be more helpful and also may decrease the risk of lightheadedness.

Although surgery was the most common treatment for BPH, many men will now proceed with medical therapy or reject surgery and accept their obstructive symptoms. Moreover, there are a variety of procedures currently being promoted (hyperthermia, microwaves, lasers) in addition to traditional transurethral resection (or in some circumstances, vaporization). The standard and most effective remains the transurethral resection (TURP). A rigid surgical instrument equipped with a microscopic lens is inserted by the surgeon through the penis into the urethra. The surgeon is thus able to view the exact spot where the prostatic urethra is being constricted and then "resect" (or cut out) the tissue judged to be causing the constriction by means of an electric loop. The prostatic urethra completely restores itself within several weeks; but, from the patient's perspective, recovery begins almost immediately. After a few days on a catheter, the patient can urinate on his own with much greater freedom from discomfort than he experienced prior to the surgery.

Although a high risk of impotence is associated with surgery for prostate cancer (i.e., a radical prostatectomy, in which the entire prostate gland is removed), TURP surgery for BPH almost never causes impotence. The nerves relating to the male erection lie on the *outside* of the prostate gland at a safe distance from the internal site of BPH development and, therefore, TURP surgery.

The few reported cases of impotence following TURP surgery have often proved to be psychological in nature.

By contrast, a common aftereffect of both kinds of surgery—TURP surgery and radical prostatectomy—is a condition called "retrograde ejaculation." Because the neck of the bladder no longer completely closes during ejaculation, the semen squirts backward into the bladder, harmlessly and imperceptibly, instead of shooting down the urethra. The "feel" of the orgasm to the patient may be just as intense and pleasurable as the feel of pre-surgery orgasms, but it will be somewhat different in kind, and the orgasm itself will be dry rather than wet (a more detailed discussion will follow in chapter 9).

Researchers have not yet established any link between BPH and prostate cancer—whether or not the BPH is treated, and, assuming it *is* treated, regardless of the particular treatment administered. But, as already mentioned, many people continue to mistake BPH for prostate cancer itself or for a precursor of prostate cancer.

One of the most infamous and intriguing cases of such a misconception concerns the British Prime Minister Harold Macmillan, an inveterate hypochondriac. In 1963, while he was still in office, he experienced acute symptoms relating to BPH and rushed into a hospital for treatment. Fearing he was only one step away from death by cancer, he told his press secretary from his hospital bed, "Of course I'm finished! I shall probably die." He resigned right away, an event that shocked the United Kingdom and precipitated a steep decline in the political fortunes of the Conservative party. A month later, to his immediate delight but later chagrin, he was feeling perfectly fit again, and he went on to live for

My Fears about BPH by Dr. Barbara

In 1979, my husband had surgery for colon cancer. We felt fortunate that the tumor was caught at an early stage and completely removed. But when a woman lives with a loved one who has had cancer—any kind of cancer—there is always a "Terror Place" in her mind, an area of fear and vigilance. If my husband starts to sleep later or has a cough that lingers longer than usual, I mentally rush to the Terror Place: the dreaded "IT" might be returning! When my husband's routine exam by a urologist indicated an enlarged prostate, or BPH, I was locked into the Terror Place.

At that time, I was extremely busy with my work. But suddenly I felt my life stand still. There was no PSA test then to help confirm or deny my fears about prostate cancer. The surgeon's office kept calling and asking my husband to make a decision one way or the other about surgery, informing him that this was "major" surgery and he could be out of commission for as long as two months. I remember standing in the kitchen one time as my husband hung up the phone after talking to the surgeon. I was frozen with fear. I felt something in my life had to give to allow me to deal with this. No matter what any doctor told us, my husband's past history of cancer loomed over us like a black cloud. I prepared immediately for the worst, cutting back my workload and professional obligations. Reason had nothing to do with it; fear—the all-consuming emotion when you're trapped in the Terror Place—simply took over.

After getting other medical opinions, my husband decided not to have surgery. Today, his BPH is an accepted part of our lives. He and our aging dogs take turns getting up at night to relieve their bladders. We stop frequently on long car trips. I don't get concerned when he stays in the men's room for what seems like forever. And yes, he has PSA and DRE tests for prostate cancer every year! However acceptable the BPH may be in our lives the fear of cancer will always be there.

another twenty-three years, dying at age ninety-three without ever having gone through another episode of prostate trouble.

Today, men who have TURP surgery, a technique that wasn't available in the United Kingdom when Macmillan suffered his health crisis, are almost always examined at the same time for prostate cancer, through a postsurgical biopsy of the tissue removed from both the prostatic urethra and the gland itself. While this biopsy is not a thorough check of the entire prostate, it's a frequent means by which early-stage, asymptomatic prostate cancers are detected.

Prostate Cancer: Why Does It Grow?

Regrettably, we know much less about why prostate cancer develops than we do about why prostatitis or BPH develops. The fact of the matter is, we know very little about why *any* type of cancer develops. For more than half of the established cancer types, including prostate cancer, no single causative agent can be specified. Among the remaining cancer types (such as lung cancer, which is known to be aggravated by smoking), many contributing causal factors are unknown in each case, so it still remains a mystery why certain established factors provoke cancer in one person and not in another.

Essentially, in *all* cancers, something goes haywire in the DNA, the basic material that encodes growth patterns within each cell, causing malformed cells to develop and multiply. Sometimes this phenomenon results in an ever-growing tumor that poses an increasing threat to normal body functions. Hence, the tumor is called "malignant," although it does not literally attack or consume healthy cells, as many laypeople think. In some cases cells from the malignant tumor break off and spread to other parts of the body, where they can spark the growth of new tumors: a process known as "metastasizing."

Prostate cancer, technically "adenocarcinoma," is classified as a "primary cancer" because it originates within the prostate gland, rather than being triggered by the invasion of cancerous cells from outside the gland. In most cases, it occurs relatively late in a man's life (usually after age fifty), starting on the rear surface of the prostate and spreading first into the gland's interior. Later, it may spread to surrounding tissues, organs, and bones, and from there to more distant areas of the body.

The cancer's rate of growth varies greatly from individual to individual; but in most cases, it grows relatively slowly. As we've already discussed in chapter 1, one in ten men eventually develops prostate cancer, but it usually doesn't manifest itself until after age fifty. Most men who live to be eighty or older have some degree of cancerous cell development inside their prostate gland; however, they typically die of other causes before any serious cancer problems arise.

Although we can't say for sure what causes prostate cancer, a number of *possible* risk factors are currently under study. Some of these possible factors are suggested by statistical evidence relating to prostate cancer patients. Other possible factors—much less substantiated and, in certain cases, purely conjectural—are based on considering the causes of other disorders that are similar in kind to prostate cancer (e.g., other types of primary cancer) or that affect the same area of the body (e.g., sexually transmitted diseases).

Discussed below are the major areas of inquiry, but first, a note of caution: Always keep in mind that *no single case of prostate cancer can yet be attributed with confidence to any particular factor or combination of factors,* so you don't want to presume to play judge, jury, or expert on your own!

Genetics

One of the most likely causes of prostate cancer is hereditary, having to do with the patient's particular genetic makeup. Statistics accumulated independently by the American Cancer Society, Medicare, and other reputable sources, all indicate that the risk of a man developing prostate cancer is doubled if his father had it, tripled if his father *and* a brother had it, and increased sixfold if his father or a brother *and* an uncle or a grandfather had it.

Another genetic question is raised by the fact that African-American men as a group have the highest rate of prostate cancer of any category of men in the world: almost 40 percent higher than Caucasian American men. By contrast Asian men have the lowest rate in the world, except for Asian men who either relocate permanently in the West (U.S. or Europe) or are born and raised in the West, in which case their rate is identical to the rate for white men in the same population area (the rate being somewhat lower for white men in Europe than white men in the U.S.).

Scientists do not yet know what to make of these contrasting rates among racial types and population areas. For example, genetics alone would not account for the increased incident rate among Asian men who move to the West. That phenomenon would seem to imply the existence of an environmental, dietary, or even lifestyle factor in prostate cancer development.

As for the comparatively high incidence among African-American men, researchers are stumped. The lower incidence of prostate cancer among black men in Africa compared to black men in the United States could be attributed to the significantly higher overall rate of prostate cancer detection and reporting in the United States compared to Africa (in all other areas of the world, "margin-of-error" adjustments are deemed more reliable). But each of these issues could be explained in many other ways as well, including ways that we aren't yet informed enough to suspect.

Statistics by themselves cannot offer proof about genetics-related issues one way or another. As soon as research identifies a specific gene related to prostate cancer (as was done in 1994 for colon cancer), scientists will be able to classify genetics as a definite developmental factor and to investigate more closely how and why this factor differs from race to race and from population area to population area.

Meanwhile, circumstantial evidence strongly suggests that all men should research their family health histories for prostate cancer, and that men with a family history of prostate cancer and all African-American men would be wise to seek early and frequent testing for prostate cancer: at least once a year after age forty.

Other genetic factors: In 1998 Dr. Michael Pollak of Montreal's McGill University, together with researchers at the Harvard School of Public Health, found that men who have elevated blood levels of a hormone called "insulin-like growth factor (IGF-1) are four times more likely to develop prostate cancer compared to those who had the lowest level of that hormone.

Diet

Studies have repeatedly indicated that a diet rich in meat and animal fats (including whole milk and ice cream) may increase the odds that a man will develop prostate cancer. Others studies aimed at establishing protective dietary factors indirectly support this hypothesis: they've found that a diet rich in beans and other vegetables appears to lower the odds. Perhaps the reason in both cases has to do with a man's testosterone level: animal foods are associated with higher testosterone production relative to vegetable foods, and testosterone is known to stimulate the growth of prostate cancer. Apart from the testosterone issue, studies of dietary factors in many other forms of cancer have also targeted a diet rich in animal fats as potentially risky.

Substance Abuse

To date, no link has been found between excessive alcohol, tobacco, or recreational drug consumption and the development of prostate cancer. Of course, substance abuse is known to have a wide range of negative effects on a person's general health and immune system capabilities, which may very well assist the growth of prostate cancer or undermine the chances for recovery from prostate cancer.

Environment

The only evidence so far regarding an environmental effect on prostate cancer development comes from studies of men who were regularly exposed, over lengthy periods of time, to cadmium, a toxic metal found in storage batteries, electroplating, and many types of metal alloys. The men in these studies had a slightly higher rate of prostate cancer than men in the general population. No definite conclusions can be drawn from these studies, but men working in jobs that involve exposure to cadmium are encouraged to seek early and frequent testing for prostate cancer.

Regarding the different rates of prostate cancer associated with the male population in different geographical areas, no definite contributing factors have been established.

Hormones

As already mentioned, the principal male hormone, testosterone, is known to stimulate the growth of prostate cancer. Whether or not it actually *starts* the development of prostate cancer has not yet been established.

Vasectomy

In February 1993 the *Journal of the American Medical Association (JAMA)* reported two studies that indicated a slightly higher risk of prostate cancer among men who have had a vasectomy, a surgical procedure that seals off the tubes carrying sperm from the testes to the urethra: one of the most effective means of contraception and one of the most common operations among adult American men (15 percent of men over age forty). An editorial accompanying the *JAMA* report recommended that men who have had vasectomies should make sure to get annual prostate checkups thereafter.

The mass media pounced on this story and the result was— and still is—a widespread misconception that the vasectomy itself creates a biological condition that increases a man's chances of developing prostate cancer. In fact, no researcher, including those who participated in the *JAMA*-reported studies, has yet established any biological reason why a vasectomy might cause a greater prostate cancer risk.

Some experts note the fact that vasectomies are sometimes followed by an increase in the production of the male hormone testosterone, a known prostate cancer stimulant. Why this happens remains a mystery, although it is often attributed to a postoperation increase in the patient's sexual activity because of his reduced fear of causing a pregnancy.

Other experts point to the fact that the men who have so far chosen to have a vasectomy do *not* represent a cross section of the U.S. male population, and therefore that other factors besides the vasectomy itself may account for the increased rate. The typical vasectomy patient, as profiled by the Association for Voluntary Surgical Contraception in New York City, is white, well educated, affluent, in his mid-to late thirties, the father of at least one son, and lives west of the Mississippi River.

In any event, other studies of a possible vasectomy-cancer link have failed to confirm the studies reported in *JAMA*. Among the most extensive of these studies was a screening of forty thousand men conducted by the urology department of the University of Colorado during Prostate Cancer Awareness Week in September 1992. According to Dr. E. David Crawford, department chairperson, "the screening detected no increase in prostate cancer rates among the estimated eight thousand participants who had undergone vasectomies."

Past Sexual Behavior

Although a man's sexual history continues to be discussed in professional circles as a potential factor in prostate cancer development, studies conducted so far offer conflicting implications. Some suggest that prostate cancer is more likely to develop in men who became sexually active at an early age and who have had many sex partners over a long period of time. If so, then a possible reason may be a consistently high level of testosterone production due to a consistently high level of sexual activity (although this explanation wouldn't take into account the issue of multiple sex partners).

Other studies point to lifelong abstinence or low sexual activity as a potential causative agent. The reasoning is that the cancer may somehow result from a buildup of testosterone within the prostate due to lack of ejaculation. Abstinence (which includes not masturbating or pursuing sexual activity to orgasm) is known to cause a discomforting backup of liquids in the prostate—a condition commonly referred to as "prostate congestion" (and less commonly dubbed "priest's disease" or "sailor's disease"). This condition clears up quickly once the pattern of abstinence is broken, something that isn't always possible for men who suffer impotence. But whether this condition can be linked to cancer is another issue entirely.

Actually, both the "high-sex" and the "low-sex" hypotheses may be true, suggesting that a *moderate* degree of sexual activity over a lifetime is the least risky course. So far, we simply don't know for sure if a man's past sexual behavior has anything at all to do with prostate cancer development.

General Lifestyle Issues

To date, no studies have shown any connection between prostate cancer development and the following general lifestyle issues:

- ◊ personality type

- ◊ emotional or situational stress

- ◊ physical exercise (or the lack thereof)

- ◊ religious affiliation or spiritual beliefs

- ◊ marital or parental status

- ◊ occupation (other than, possibly, in the metalworking industries: see "Environment" earlier in this chapter)

Men who are economically deprived, or who have a relatively poor educational background, do have a higher rate of advanced-stage prostate cancer; but most experts attribute this to the fact that men in these categories are also less likely to seek medical testing or intervention until their illness is well advanced and physically hard to endure.

Prostate Cancer: How Does It Develop?

Traditionally, urologists have divided prostate cancer development into four basic stages, beginning with the easiest to treat, which was labeled Stage A/T1, and progressing on through Stages B/T2 and C/T3 or T4 to the most advanced and most difficult to treat Stage D/N+ or M+. Recently this nomenclature has changed. Because the system is still in transition, we will use the traditional system throughout this book but include the following chart to allow you to compare the two.

Old System	New System	Characteristics
A	T1	Confined to prostate but not detectable by digital rectal examination or ultrasound: detected unexpectedly
B	T2	Confined to prostate; detected by digital rectal examination or ultrasound
C	T3 or T4	Locally advanced beyond prostate
D	N+	Spread to lymph nodes (N+)
	M+	Spread to distant organs

Treatment decisions are based on the developmental stage of a patient's cancer, so it's important to understand the basic stage-related characteristics (for information on the particular treatments most often prescribed for each stage, see chapter 6, "Choosing among Treatment Options"). Also, bear in mind that, in some situations, two slightly different stage classifications may be applied to the same cancer. For example, a cancer that is "clinically" designated Stage C/T3 or T4 (based on the clinical definition of that stage) may be "pathologically" designated Stage D/N+ or M+ (based on the illness that the patient is apparently experiencing).

Stage A/T1

A Stage A/T1 prostate cancer is confined to the prostate gland itself and is microscopically small—too small to be detected by a digital rectal examination (in which the examining doctor's finger is inserted up the rectum to feel for hard or "bumpy" cancerous tissue on the prostate).

A patient can have Stage A/T1 cancer for years without feeling any symptoms. Until recently, Stage A/T1 cancer was rarely detected, except in cases where a pathologic examination was performed on prostate tissue obtained during surgery for benign prostate enlargement (BPH). Now, the existence of Stage A/T1 cancer can also be detected through a PSA (prostate-specific antigen) test of a blood sample, as already discussed in chapter 1, and as further described in chapter 3.

Stage A/T1 cancer is subdivided into two categories: Stage A/T1 and Stage A/T2. In Stage A/Tl cancer, no more than 5 percent of the tissue examined in the biopsy consists of cancerous cells. In Stage A/T2 cancer, more than 5 percent of the tissue is cancerous. In comparing stage A/T1 with A/T2 disease, another distinction is the higher grade of the latter and its greater potential for progression. Therefore, treatment choice would best be made on ten and fifteen year survival time rather than five year survival time. According to the American Cancer Society, over 95 percent of men who are treated for Stage A/T1 cancer (both subdivisions combined) are alive after five years.

Stage B/T2

Stage B/T2 cancer features a tumor that has not yet spread beyond the prostate gland itself, but is big enough to be felt in a digital rectal exam (although it can still be missed due to the relatively crude nature of the exam). If a urologist does feel a suspicious hardness or bump in the prostate, indicating the possibility of a tumor, he or she usually orders a PSA test and, if warranted, a biopsy. At least 40 percent of prostatectomy specimens clinically staged as B/T2 are found to have penetrated the capsule. Extensive penetration is associated with treatment failure.

A patient with Stage B/T2 cancer may not feel any symptoms. If he does, they most often involve urinary problems, such as frequent urination, hesitancy during urination, thinner-than-normal stream, or attacks of atypical urgency. These symptoms are also characteristic of benign prostate enlargement (BPH). When a patient complains of them, a urologist usually orders a PSA test, and possibly a biopsy, to determine whether the cause is BPH or cancer.

Stage B/T2 cancer is subdivided into three categories: Stages Bl, B2, and B3. In Stage B2, the tumor is located in only one lobe (of two) in the prostate and is less than one centimeter (approximately one half of an inch) in diameter. In Stage B2, the tumor is larger than two centimeters in diameter, involving almost the entire lobe. In Stage B3, the cancer has spread through both lobes of the prostate (in some instances where the cancer has spread to both lobes, but does not form a very large total, it is designated Stage B2 rather than B3). According to the American Cancer Society, 85 percent of men treated for Stage B/T2 cancer—all three subdivisions combined—survive beyond five years.

Stage C/T3 or T4

In Stage C/T3 or C/T4 cancer, the malignant tumor has grown beyond the muscular casing of the prostate gland into the immediately surrounding tissue. It has not yet advanced into the lymph glands, but it may have spread into the seminal vesicles, the semen-producing glands that lie just above the rear of the prostate.

Stage C/T3 or C/T4 cancer is subdivided into two categories: Cl and C2. In Stage C1 cancer, the cancer has just begun to spread outside the prostate gland and the tumor remains comparatively small. The patient may or may not feel any symptoms. The larger size of the Stage C2 tumor can't help but cause significant pressure on the urethra, which almost always produces mild pain in the upper groin and pronounced urinary problems (more discomforting than the potential Stage B problems mentioned earlier).

A Stage C/T3 or C/T4 tumor is easily detectable during a digital rectal exam. If the urologist suspects that the cancer is this far evolved, he or she is likely to order an ultrasound exam, a prostatic acid phosphatase (PAP) test, biopsies of tissues surrounding the prostate gland, and/or bone marrow tests to determine more precisely just how far advanced the cancer is (see chapter 3 for descriptions of these tests). According to the American Cancer Society, almost 70 percent of men who are treated for Stage C/T3 or C/T4 cancer are alive after five years.

Stage D/N+ or M+

A Stage D/N+ or M+ cancer is one in which the original tumor has metastasized, spreading the cancer beyond the area immediately surrounding the prostate gland to the lymph nodes and possibly to other parts of the body, including the bones, bladder, liver, and/or lungs. Depending upon how far advanced the Stage D/N+ or M+ cancer is, the patient may or may not experience obvious problems in voiding. More severe symptoms—like ongoing pain in the body's midsection, noticeable weight loss, and a general malaise—usually occur only in cases of very advanced Stage D/N+ or M+ cancer.

Stage D/N+ or M+ cancer is subdivided into four categories: D0, Dl, D2, and D3. These categories are defined as follows:

◊ D0: High-reading enzyme tests suggest that the cancer has reached Stage D/N+ or M+, but there are no other indications.

◊ Dl: Cancer is detected in the lymph nodes close by the prostate gland.

◊ D2: Cancer is detected in the lymph nodes and in other parts of the body beyond the area immediately surrounding the prostate.

◊ D3: Not used in the diagnosis itself, the classification D3 includes former D2 cancers that were treated but nevertheless continued to spread.

To determine the presence and extent of a single case of Stage D/N+ or M+ cancer, urologists may use a number of different diagnostic procedures, including blood tests, X-rays, computerized tomography (CT), magnetic resonance imaging (MRI), a pyelogram, and/or a bone scan, followed by biopsies of suspected tissues. For more information on these tests, see chapter 3. The American Cancer Society estimates that less than 30 percent of men treated for Stage D/N+ or M+ cancer (all subdivisions combined) are alive five years later, pointing to a dramatic decrease in the effectiveness of treatment for Stage D/N+ or M+ cancer as compared to Stage C/T3 or T4 cancer (which has a five year survival rate of almost 70 percent). This fact alone underscores the importance of seeking testing and treatment for prostate cancer sooner rather than later.

3

Detection and Diagnosis

◊ Physical symptoms that may be caused by prostate cancer

◊ Questions to ask your doctor about testing

◊ Common diagnostic tests performed to verify
prostate cancer and its extent

For once, the medical and journalistic worlds agree: Prostate cancer deserves to be called "the silent killer." A man is not likely to
experience tangible symptoms of prostate cancer's existence until
it is relatively well advanced (i.e., Stage B/T2 or Stage C/T3 or
T4). Even then, the symptoms usually remain mild enough to
tolerate—and ignore—for months or even years.

By the time that prostate cancer symptoms become alarm-
ingly strong or incapacitating (Stage D/N+ or M+), the cancer has
usually evolved to the point that it's almost sure to cause the

patient's death within two to three years if it isn't treated. Even with treatment, only about 50 percent of patients will survive beyond this time period. And there isn't always a warning signal. Often prostate cancer reaches this life-threatening level without causing severe symptoms.

Granted, the latter situation is a worst-case scenario: Most men who develop prostate cancer die of other, unrelated causes before their prostate cancer ever becomes far enough advanced to cause serious symptoms. Nevertheless, for the man over forty, this very scary, worst case scenario warrants paying especially close attention to any of the physical symptoms listed below. The symptom may indicate prostatitis or an enlarged prostate: far more common disorders than prostate cancer. But it may—in addition or instead—signify prostate cancer, a potential killer beginning to break its silence.

Possible Symptoms of Prostate Cancer

◊ a weaker-than-normal urinary flow (a thinner, slower stream of urine with less of an "arc" than before)

◊ repeated difficulty in starting a urinary flow (technically called "hesitancy")

◊ recurring episodes of interruptions in the urinary flow (involuntary stops and starts) or "failed" urinations (inability to produce a urinary flow, despite desire and pressure)

◊ greater-than-normal frequency of urination

◊ a pattern of being awakened several times during the course of nighttime sleep by the need to urinate, technically called "nocturia"

◊ greater-than-normal urinary dribbling after completing urination

◊ recurring times when the bladder doesn't feel completely empty, even after urinating as much as possible

- episodes of an overwhelming pressure to urinate at inappropriate times (technically called "urgency," this situation occurs inexplicably, i.e., when the bladder has *not* been overly challenged by liquid intake or by a lengthy period of time since the last urination)

- painful urination (technically called "dysuria") or painful ejaculation: both usually felt as a burning or "ripping" sensation in the penis

- inability to control urination (technically called "incontinence," which could include occasional episodes of bedwetting)

- blood in the urine or semen

- dull, inexplicable pain in the pelvis, hips, lower back, kidneys, or thighs that lasts for longer than two weeks without interruption

When any one of these symptoms persists for two or more months, and especially when any combination of these symptoms persists for that long, a man should inform his partner and then consult with a urologist, asking specifically for prostate cancer testing.

Because of the small size of the prostate gland and its intricate, deeply internal placement in the male anatomy, it is notoriously difficult to examine. Add to this fact the mysterious nature of prostate cancer itself—with its unknown causes, lack of clear-cut symptoms, and unpredictable growth pattern—and the result is a host of different medical tests and techniques that are utilized on a step-by-step basis to answer different kinds of questions. Among those questions are (in order of inquiry):

1. Is there any reason to believe that prostate cancer *may* be present, even though there are no *definitive* symptoms and it can't be felt by the examining urologist?

2. Is prostate cancer *actually* present?

3. How far has the prostate cancer already advanced (i.e., what *stage* is this cancer and to what areas has it spread)?

4. At what rate, and to what areas, is this particular prostate
cancer likely to develop in the future?

As we've already discussed, the potential value of annual
prostate cancer testing for men over age fifty—or over age forty
for African-Americans and men with a family history of prostate
cancer—is enormous. The current five-year survival rate among
patients treated for Stages A/T1 and B/T2 prostate cancers (both
categories combined) is close to 90 percent, compared to a 50 percent rate of surviving less than three years among men treated for
more advanced Stages C/T3 or T4 and D/N+ or M+ cancers (both
categories combined).

True, the issue of how soon, or how aggressively, to treat
early-stage prostate cancer has now become very controversial,
thanks to the earlier and easier detection of the cancer's presence
made possible by the PSA (prostate-specific antigen) blood test.
But treatment-related issues should not be confused with
diagnosis-related issues. To avoid diagnosis and therefore to
remain ignorant about the possible presence of prostate cancer
may be a way to avoid the treatment-related controversy, but it is
hardly an intelligent way. Indeed, it can be disastrous.

Difficult as it may be for a man and his mate to live with the
knowledge that the man has prostate cancer, and to make—or
postpone—treatment decisions based on this knowledge, the possible alternative is much worse. They may not discover that the
man has prostate cancer until it's too late to do much about it, and
they may then come to the realization that either of them might
have prevented this tragedy from happening with just a little
more common sense and courage at an earlier time in their lives.

Regardless of whether a man's prostate cancer is detected
early or late in its development, the process of arriving at a precise and reliable diagnosis can be long, arduous, and bewildering
to him and his caregiver, leading them from doctor to doctor, and
test to test. New investigative procedures may have to be
performed—or former ones repeated—at any time in the course of
the illness: to confirm or refine a diagnosis, to gauge the effectiveness of a treatment under progress, to investigate a new finding
during treatment, or to check for posttreatment complications or
resurgencies.

Both your partner and you, his caregiver, need to prepare yourselves to ask the right questions and to understand the answers you are given at any time when prostate cancer testing occurs—from the initial diagnosis to the posttreatment checkups. The basic questions you should ask are these:

Questions to Ask about Prostate Cancer Tests

Why is this test being ordered?

◊ What circumstances warrant it?

◊ What is it expected to accomplish?

◊ How important is it in diagnosing and treating the patient's condition?

How will this test be performed?

◊ Where will it be performed?

◊ Who will perform it?

◊ What is the basic procedure for the test?

◊ How, specifically, might the test itself affect the patient (physical discomfort, time spent, possible aftereffects)?

◊ Are there ways that possible negative effects can be prevented, minimized, or managed?

What does the test cost?

◊ Is the cost covered by his/my/our insurance?

◊ Are there any options that might affect the cost? For example, would it be less expensive to have the test performed in a clinic rather than in a private lab?

◊ Is there any possibility that unforeseen developments might make the test cost more than the original quote?

When and how will we know the results?

◊ When is the earliest/latest time that the results might be available?

◊ Would you please contact us personally with the results?

(NOTE: Ideally, you and the patient should be informed *jointly* about the results by the doctor who is ordering the test, so that he or she can immediately respond to any questions that you have about the actual meaning of the results in terms of this particular case.)

◊ *How useful would other kinds of tests be?*
This is a question that should be posed at least two times for every test that is ordered:

1. when the test is first recommended (in case, for example, another test could be administered at the same time as, or instead of, the recommended one); and

2. when the results of that test are announced (in case, for example, another test might yield additional information that would help you to make a difficult treatment decision).

At each of these times, use the list of major diagnostic tests in this chapter, as well as any other test-related data that you obtain, to ask your doctor the following questions about every other test that seems relevant to the situation:

◊ Would this test [named by you] be helpful?

◊ If so, how?

◊ If not, why?

Don't be afraid to seek second or third opinions about the possible merits of specific tests from other doctors as well. Ask your doctor (and/or other reliable sources) for the names of other doctors who are knowledgeable about the tests involved.

Common Tests for Detecting and Diagnosing Prostate Cancer

Described below are the tests that doctors most commonly perform or request in order to detect or diagnose prostate cancer.

These descriptions, combined with data from your own independent research, will prepare you not only to ask doctors appropriate questions about different kinds of prostate cancer tests but also to understand the test-related information and results that doctors give you. (For questions to ask your doctor *after* prostate cancer has been initially diagnosed, see chapter 4.)

Common Diagnostic Tests

Test	Description
Digital Rectal Exam (DRE)	Finger inserted in anus probes for suspicious prostate lumps
Prostate-Specific Antigen (PSA)	Blood test: level of PSA rises if prostate cancer present
Transrectal Ultrasound (TRUS)	Device inserted in rectum makes sound-wave picture of prostate
Biopsy	Surgery: sample of prostate tissue is removed and examined

Less Common Diagnostic Tests

Test	Description
Intravenous Pyelogram (IVP)*†	X-ray of kidneys, bladder, and ureter after dye injection
Bone Scan injection*	X-ray of bones after dye
Chest X-ray*	X-ray of lungs
Computed Tomography (CT)**	Computerized X-ray of midsection
Magnetic Resonance Imaging (MRI)**	Computer images of midsection subjected to magnetic field

---

*   checks for cancer spread beyond prostate
†   Intravenous Pyelogram is used in advanced prostate cancer in which ureteral obstructrion may be found
** checks for cancer confined to, or spread beyond, prostate

Common Testing Pattern

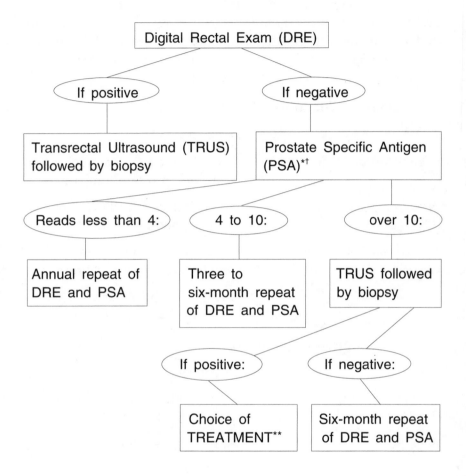

---

* Very often this is done regardless of the results of the DRE or whether or not the DRE is omitted.

† A PSA reading <4 ng/ml may indicate the need for transrectal ultrasound/biopsy if the reading is higher than one would suspect for a particular patient's age, or if there is a strong family history of prostate cancer. A PSA reading of 4–10 ng/ml might prompt a repeat evaluation at three months, especially if there has been a lower level previously.

** Even if a biopsy is positive, treatment might not be chosen either on account of the patient's own desires, the finding of a low grade malignancy, or a patient's age/concomitant medical conditions.

Digital Rectal Examination (DRE)

The rear of the prostate gland, where prostate cancer is most likely to start developing, can be felt by touch through the tissue lining a man's rectum, at a point about two and a half inches up the rectum pressing frontward, toward the pubic bone. In a digital rectal exam (DRE), the doctor inserts a lubricated gloved finger into the rectum and probes gently across the rear of the prostate gland to determine whether there is any hardened—i.e., cancerous—tissue.

To get an idea of how normal, noncancerous prostate tissue feels to the examining doctor, place your index finger lightly on the tip of your nose and push gently against the tissue there. It should feel slightly spongy. Now, to get an idea of how hardened, cancerous tissue feels by comparison, place your index finger lightly against the middle of your forehead and push gently against the tissue there. It should feel relatively hard. In addition to feeling hard, prostate cancer tissue may also feel somewhat corrugated (normal prostate tissue feels smooth).

The DRE is not a very precise examination. It can miss certain cancers that are too small, that are atypically located on the *front* surface of the prostate, or that are engulfed by noncancerous tissue due to prostate enlargement (BPH). However, the testing procedure itself is quick, easy, and fairly painless, although a bit uncomfortable. For decades, until the development of the PSA test, the DRE was the principal means of determining whether or not a man should undergo more sophisticated prostate cancer tests, and it remains a very important first-step investigatory procedure.

According to the American Cancer Society, the DRE should be part of an annual rectal exam for *all* men over age fifty—a comprehensive exam that checks not only for prostate cancer, but also for rectal cancer, which can manifest itself earlier in a man's lifetime. Regrettably, the DRE is still far from being the standard procedure it should be for *any* man in this age group who undergoes a routine physical.

Surveys have repeatedly shown that many men, unaccustomed to having their bodies probed and, in some cases, overly sensitized by homophobia, dread the mere idea of having another person—even a doctor—place a finger into the anus. Some men are so disturbed by this possibility that they won't ask for the test themselves, won't mention symptoms that might lead to it, or even go to a doctor in the first place. Alternatively, many doctors, well aware of such feelings, are reluctant to perform the exam, unless the patient specifically requests it or there is other evidence of possible prostate cancer. The sad result of this "DRE-phobia" is many cases of advanced prostate cancer that could have been detected and treated at a much earlier stage.

Prostate-Specific Antigen Test (PSA)

Before we begin a discussion of the PSA, it should be emphasized that PSA is a "prostate-specific" marker and not a "prostate cancer-specific" marker. The influence of benign enlargement of the prostate, inflammation, infection, and trauma can effect the levels of PSA in the absence of malignancy. In the PSA the patient's blood is analyzed in a laboratory to determine the level of a protein—or antigen—that is only produced by the prostate gland. Researchers aren't sure what this protein does. They think it may help the semen maintain a liquid consistency. What they do know for sure is that when a problem occurs in the prostate, the blood sample may show a higher-than-normal level of this protein—up to ten times the normal amount. The reason the bloodstream contains a higher level of PSA is that it is leaking more profusely out of the problematic prostate tissue. The problem itself might be prostatitis, benign prostate hyperplasia (BPH), or prostate cancer. Progressive elevation of this level over time (detected by periodic testing) suggests that the problem—whatever it may be—is worsening and gives some indication of the rate of spread.

Generally, a prostate-specific antigen (PSA) count below 4 ng/ml (indicating nanograms, or billionths of a gram, per milliliter of blood) is considered normal. If a patient's PSA count registers between 4 and 10, his estimated chances of having prostate cancer, as opposed to another, less serious problem, range from 20 to 50 percent (estimates vary from expert to expert, although all estimates rise as the count rises). If his PSA count goes above 10, the chances are 50 to 75 percent; above 20, over 90 percent.

As definitive as the PSA test sounds, it has its problems. Sometimes, from the perspective of screening for possible prostate cancer, the test gives "false positives," i.e., high counts that are *not* associated with cancerous tissue. In certain cases, the factor causing this high count can be established; as already mentioned, prostatitis and BPH may be prompting greater PSA leakage. In other cases, the factor causing the false positive may remain a mystery. Conversely, the PSA count can be kept misleadingly *low* by certain factors: some known (for example, the drug Proscar, commonly prescribed for the treatment of BPH); others unknown.

For these reasons, the best way to use the PSA test as a diagnostic tool is in combination with other tests, such as the DRE or transrectal ultrasound. Another approach is to consider the first PSA reading as a "base-level" count, and then go on to track PSA readings over two-month, three-month, six-month, or one-year intervals, depending on the apparent gravity of the situation. Any PSA level that rises more than .75 ng/ml over the course of a year of testing indicates a seriously worsening condition—possibly involving prostate cancer, prostatitis, or BPH. The periodic-testing approach is especially advisable for men whose initial reading falls within the "normal" to "low-risk" range. It may be inappropriately conservative for a patient who appears to be at higher risk.

Since 1992 the American Cancer Society began recommending an annual PSA test for all men over age fifty (over age forty for African-Americans and men with a family history of prostate cancer). On August 29, 1994, after years of internal debate, the PSA test was approved for diagnostic use by the federal Food and Drug Administration (FDA), with the stipulation that it should always be administered in conjunction with the DRE. The validity of this recommendation remains controversial. Unfortunately we're still unable to distinguish between those cancers that will be clinically significant and those that are not, and never will be, clinically significant. Some men will die *with* prostate cancer, not *because* of prostate cancer.

Some health-care providers suggest that PSA testing for the older person in the absence of a positive digital rectal examination is unnecessary, so you may need to determine for yourself what "older" means.

Transrectal Ultrasound (TRUS)

The transrectal ultrasound (TRUS) test, often referred to as "ultrasound imaging" or a "sonogram," works like underwater sonar does in a battleship or submarine. While the patient lies fully conscious on his side or back, a slender device called a transducer (actually a probe covered by a water-filled balloon) is inserted into the rectum next to the prostate gland. For approximately fifteen minutes, during which the patient feels only the mild discomfort of having the slim, soft instrument three inches up his rectum, the transducer bounces high-frequency sound waves off the prostate gland. As the waves return, it relays them to an outside sensing machine that translates them into a detailed visual image of the gland: first, on a screen; later, on a film sheet. Hopefully, any cancerous tissue will show up in this image, because sound waves travel at different rates through tissues of different densities.

A TRUS test can be very effective in discovering tumors that are not detected by a DRE. It can also help determine whether a high PSA test result is due to BPH or prostate cancer. The one major drawback associated with TRUS is that it often gives indeterminate or false readings (either positive or negative). Researchers are now seeking ways to improve the quality and accuracy of TRUS-produced images.

Cystoscopy

The doctor carefully inserts a thin, lubricated viewing instrument into the penis and up through the urethra, looking for evidence that the prostate gland has grown and, in doing so, has adversely affected the urethra lining. Usually performed to examine bladder problems or to diagnose benign prostate enlargement

(BPH), the cystoscopy is not considered by some doctors to be a necessary test for detecting prostate cancer; but others—including those who have had a great deal of experience with it—find it worthwhile. The procedure is not as painful for the patient as it sounds, but it can be uncomfortable. Fortunately, the test only takes a minute or two to perform.

Biopsy

A biopsy of the prostate gland is a relatively minor surgical procedure in which a small amount of tissue is extracted from a suspected area of the prostate gland itself (or, in later biopsies for more advanced cancers, other parts of the body) and then examined under a microscope for the presence of cancerous cells. It is almost always performed if the DRE, PSA test, and/or TRUS test indicate that prostate cancer may be present.

The biopsy can be performed in a number of different ways, according to what the doctor deems advisable in consultation with the patient. Most doctors today use a spring-loaded needle "gun" that is inserted into the rectum so that the needle can collect samples from the prostate by passing through the adjacent rectal lining. Often the needle gun is used in conjunction with an ultrasound probe, which helps to target suspect areas of the prostate for the needle to hit.

The gun-plus-ultrasound biopsy sounds more uncomfortable to the patient than it actually is. Both instruments are slender, and the rectal lining has relatively few nerve endings to register pain. Whether or not the needle gun is accompanied by an ultrasound probe, the procedure can often be done without any anesthesia, and it normally lasts less than ten minutes.

Another biopsy procedure involves a very thin needle inserted through the perineum, the space on a man's body between the anus and the scrotum. There's also a thin-needle, transrectal technique called "fine-needle aspiration cytology," in which a very fine needle "sucks" rather than scrapes cells from different spots on the prostate, thus minimizing bleeding and any chance of infection. Again, these techniques usually require no anesthesia.

Finally, there are the transrectal biopsies that use larger needles, including the so-called "core needle," which is approximately the diameter of pencil lead and which necessitates the use of a local anesthetic or (in some cases) a spinal or general anesthetic. These larger needle biopsies obtain larger tissue samples, which many doctors believe are more reliable. Sometimes the doctor will order a larger-needle biopsy if the results of a thin needle biopsy are ambiguous.

If a biopsy reveals cancer cells, the doctor goes on to "grade" the tumor, assessing through personal judgment the cancer's *stage* of growth (A through D, D being the most evolved: see chapter 2) and giving it a *Gleason score* from 2 to 10 (indicating how aggressively the cancer appears to be developing, based on the cell structure: 10 being the most aggressive rating). Sometimes, the doctor orders a *ploidy analysis* of the cancerous cells, a very sophisticated and expensive test that examines their genetic makeup and grades it from 1 (lowest grade of malignancy) to 4 (highest grade).

After evaluating a biopsy that reveals cancerous cells, the doctor often orders additional tests to determine more about the cancer's extent and aggressiveness. The results of these tests may require an adjustment of the original, postbiopsy grading of the cancer. If the biopsy does *not* reveal cancer cells, the doctor may schedule another biopsy of the prostate gland for several months later, just to make sure.

A special kind of biopsy, called a *pelvic node dissection* or *lymphadenectomy*, is performed on tissue taken from the pelvic lymph nodes to determine if prostate cancer has spread that far. Usually, the tissue is obtained during the course of surgery to remove a cancerous prostate gland (i.e., a radical prostatectomy).

A new microsurgical approach to pelvic node dissection involves inserting a viewing-and-cutting instrument (technically called a "laparoscope") through an incision into the abdomen to remove samples of any suspicious lymph node tissue for study. This approach entails very little pain or discomfort for the patient, who, in most cases, spends less than twenty-four hours in the hospital. Women commonly undergo a similar form of laparoscopy for exploratory purposes or for tubal ligation.

Intravenous Pyelogram (IVP)

Today, most doctors believe that an intravenous pyelogram is unnecessary to test for possible prostate cancer. Therefore, if your doctor recommends an IVP, be sure to bring up this fact, and ask him or her for more explanation regarding why the IVP is being suggested, as opposed to another, more commonly used test that can achieve the same purpose.

As for how the IVP test works, a radioactive dye specifically designed for the IVP is injected into the patient's bloodstream, usually through the forearm. After the dye has had time to permeate the kidney, ureter, and bladder tissues, a number of X-rays are taken of these areas over a period of about one half hour to determine if cancer has infiltrated.

The IVP is a relatively arduous procedure, and some patients may suffer serious allergic reactions to the dye. For many years, the IVP and the lymphangiogram (a similar test that is now no longer performed for prostate cancer diagnosis) were the only ways to visualize possible cancerous areas in this part of the body without performing exploratory surgery. Now we have other techniques that are easier, more comfortable for the patient, less expensive, and, in many cases, able to satisfy all the needs of the situation. They include transrectal ultrasound (TRUS), (described earlier) for early, less comprehensive investigations; and computed tomography (CT) or magnetic resonance imaging (MRI), (described later in this chapter), for more thorough investigations.

Bone Scan

A radioactive dye specifically designed for the bone scan is injected into the bloodstream, usually through the arm, and allowed to filter into the bones (which takes around twenty-four hours). An X-ray then reveals "defects" in bone structure that may be due to cancer.

A major drawback of the bone scan is the fact that it doesn't detect the presence of cancer itself, but rather the presence of damaged tissue. Instead of cancer, the defects revealed by the test may have been caused by fracturing, arthritis, or any one of a number of bacterial infections. However, if the existence of prostate cancer in the patient's body has already been established, and if the bone damage appears fairly extensive—especially in the spine, the pelvis, the hips, and/or the upper legs—then the odds are high that the bone damage was caused by cancer.

Chest X-Ray

A standard, painless chest X-ray (no dye injection needed) helps the doctor determine whether cancerous tissue has evolved in the lungs. The spread of prostate cancer to the lungs is a relatively rare development associated with late-stage cancers, but sometimes a doctor orders a chest X-ray in any case, just to be on the safe side, especially if the patient has not had one in a long time (a chest X-ray should be part of a routine annual checkup for men over fifty).

Computed Tomography (CT)

During a computed tomography (CT) scan for possible prostate cancer, the patient lies still on a flat surface, with his body's midsection ringed vertically, in "doughnut" fashion, by a scanning mechanism. A rotating X-ray beam, housed in this scanning mechanism, takes a series of pictures of the interior of the patient's midsection from a range of different angles. A computer renders these pictures into cross-section "slice images" that show varying densities of tissues. The doctor then examines these images to determine if any densities are indicative of cancer: not only in the prostate gland but also in surrounding areas.

On the positive side, a CT scan frequently helps doctors determine whether prostate cancer has spread to the lymph nodes, the liver, the bladder, or the kidneys. On the negative side, it is relatively expensive (around $500-$800 on the average) and the images it produces, especially in cases of early-stage prostate cancer, are often not precise enough to indicate much beyond prostate enlargement—although this in itself can be very helpful information. Sometimes patients are injected with a special dye prior to a CT scan that might be able to enhance the image quality. It is hoped that technical refinements in the near future will make the CT scan significantly more effective in diagnosing prostate cancer.

Magnetic Resonance Imaging (MRI)

The magnetic resonance imaging (MRI) procedure represents a big step beyond the CT scan in visual quality. The patient, lying on a flat surface, is inserted completely inside a tubelike chamber that functions as a large circular electromagnet, generating a magnetic field that prompts electrical charges from the patient's body. These charges are picked up by a sensor and computer-translated into images that are much clearer and more detailed than CT pictures. The procedure is painless and safe; and, when the images can be read as cancer-related with a high degree of confidence (sometimes they can't), they can be invaluable aids in making treatment decisions.

Unfortunately, the MRI procedure also represents a giant step beyond the CT scan in expense and discomfort. It can easily cost over $1,000; and many patients experience claustrophobia or even anxiety attacks during the lengthy time (forty-five minutes to an hour on the average) that they have to spend motionless inside the MRI chamber. For these reasons, it isn't used very often in prostate cancer diagnosis unless special circumstances appear to warrant it. Future technical improvements may make it a more helpful, and more patient friendly, tool.

In the meantime, if an MRI is required and the patient is concerned about whether or not he can tolerate the procedure, ask the doctor for help in locating the least confining MRI technology within the area in which you're willing—or able—to travel. Also, tranquilizers and/or psychological interventions such as hypnosis can be very helpful.

4

Dealing with the Diagnosis: Practical Matters

◊ How to start gathering and evaluating information about prostate cancer

◊ How to question the doctor about the diagnosis

◊ How to determine if the doctor is right for the patient

◊ How to inform others about the diagnosis

Each man reacts to a diagnosis of prostate cancer in his own way, as each woman reacts to a man's diagnosis in her own way. And yet they all share the experience of entering a strange new world of turmoil and anguish, both for themselves as individuals and for their relationships. Let's begin exploring this world by considering the reactions of three different couples to a diagnosis of prostate cancer.

Tom, age 50, and Rebecca, age 45

Tom was told by his doctor to bring Rebecca to a meeting about his prostate tests. "I knew then that my worst fears had come true," he remembered, "but that inner knowledge didn't help. When he told me about my cancerous situation, he seemed to be speaking to something or someone at a point over my head. The calm, crisp evenness of his voice made the report even harder to bear than I had imagined. I just couldn't think. All I could do for a long time was moan, groan, and jabber."

Rebecca, by contrast, was suffering a gamut of thoughts and emotions. "My husband had always been a very active, good, capable man, and I ached unbearably for him. This made the urgency of everything very hard to take. I knew, suddenly, that I was going to have to be in charge in a way I hadn't been in our entire marriage. My mood kept swinging from disbelief to fatalism. It was exhausting. Just when Tom needed my help most, I felt that I needed help myself."

Allen, age 59, and Kate, age 39

Allen was hospitalized for a kidney stone when he heard that a biopsy of his prostate tissue was "positive," specifically "four plus three, which is seven on a scale of one to ten." He was exasperated. The words had no meaning to him. Finally, he heard the doctor say *cancer*, and, in Allen's own words, "It was like I'd been living inside a magic bubble before, and now that bubble had burst." His first response was shock, which slowly gave way to anger. "I was mad at the world for what happened to me," he said. Partly to punish the world, and partly just to keep the anger from showing, he withdrew into silence.

Meanwhile, Kate was extremely agitated by the news, and desperate for reassurance. She was considerably younger than Allen, and they had only been married a year and a half. Now the "verdict," as her husband had called the diagnosis, seemed at times like a judgment against the logic of their brave, freshly forged relationship. "I was flipping out," she recalled, "and the worst of it was, I didn't know who to talk to."

Leonard, age 63, and Joanne, age 60

Following treatment for a concussion, Leonard still wasn't feeling well, so he went to the doctor for a complete physical. This led to a prostate biopsy. When he phoned his doctor's office later to ask about the biopsy results, his nurse said over the phone, "You have CA." "You mean cancer?" he asked. "Yes," she replied. Later, he recalled, "It was funny: I think I was so put off by the clumsy way I was told about it, that I didn't have much response to the news itself. When it did hit me, I said to myself, *Stop! It will be okay. I'll get rid of the cancer. Nothing's going to happen to me.* I did everything I could to put it out of my mind."

Joanne, also, was distressed by the way she heard the news. "Leonard simply hung up the phone and said, 'Well, it's malignant, but it's no big deal.' I was totally floored. This just kept being his attitude, and I just kept getting angrier and angrier. He wasn't taking it as seriously as I thought he should, especially since we'd always been so close. I'd say to myself, *This is his life, and he's a big boy, but this affects me too!*"

The responses of these individuals to a diagnosis of prostate cancer vary greatly. Among the men, they range from an apparent absence of emotion ("No big deal") to a host of overwhelming emotions ("My worst fears come true"); from diffidence ("Nothing's going to happen to me") to defiant rage ("Mad at the world for what's happened to me"). Among the women, there's a similarly broad spectrum of responses, from panic ("I was flipping out") to collapse ("It was exhausting"); from deep compassion ("I ached unbearably for him") to intense frustration ("I just kept getting angrier and angrier").

Nevertheless, listening to these responses, we hear strong common chords. No one—victim or partner—is ever quite prepared for confronting a diagnosis of prostate cancer, regardless of how much that diagnosis has been anticipated. Everyone seeks to have control over his or her automatic reactions, which are too disturbing to tolerate, but this is impossible given the shocking nature of the news. And everyone, no matter how intimately involved in a partnership he or she may be, suddenly feels very much alone.

Unfortunately, this crisis of feeling suffered by both individuals comes at a time in the illness when they are most called upon to be rational, resourceful, and energetic in attending to pragmatic matters. With this in mind, let's look first at what a couple needs to do on a *practical* level, immediately after the diagnosis. Later, in chapter 5, we'll examine how each person can better handle the *emotional* issues that arise immediately after the diagnosis—issues that can come and go, or linger, throughout the course of the illness.

The four main areas of practical concern immediately after diagnosis are:

1. gathering and evaluating information about prostate cancer

2. talking with the doctor about the diagnosis

3. determining if the doctor is right for the patient

4. informing others about the diagnosis

Each of these areas is discussed below.

1. Gathering and Evaluating Information about Prostate Cancer.

For Immediate Action

After finding out from your doctor how soon you need to make a treatment decision:

⬥ Call the National Cancer Institute, 1-800-4-CANCER, and ask for information about prostate cancer.

⬥ Call Us Too, a patient support group, 1-800-80-US-TOO, and ask for information about support groups.

⬥ Call AACT (Patient Advocates for Advanced Cancer Treatments), 1-616-453-3147 (Grand Rapids, Michigan), and ask for information about prostate cancer.

⬥ Call your local chapter of the American Cancer Society (or the national organization, 1-800-ACS-2345) and ask what services they can offer you.

Although your doctor may remain your *primary* source of information about prostate cancer, he or she should not be your *only* source. Despite the emotional shock or upheaval you may be experiencing, you need to begin tapping a variety of different information sources right away, not only so that you can become more fully informed about the illness, treatment options, and patient/caretaker assistance possibilities but also so that you can more objectively assess the quality of care you're receiving from your doctor. It may help to keep a notebook in which you can record questions and leads that you want to pursue as well as contact data that you accumulate (names, addresses, phone numbers, and directions).

The first step in your independent research should be to call the numbers listed above, "For Immediate Action," and ask for the most up-to-date pamphlets, reports, and other information that they can send you relative to your particular situation. When contacting patient support groups like Us Too, Man to Man, or PAACT (Patient Advocates for Advanced Cancer Treatments), describe as specifically as you can what you know about your diagnosis so far, and ask for the names and telephone numbers of members who had similar diagnoses and who would be willing to talk with you about their experiences with prostate cancer. (For more contact information, see the "Resources" section in chapter 10.)

Then, ask your local librarian about the most recent and authoritative material in the library concerning prostate cancer. If you are fortunate enough to live in a city with a medical library, do not hesitate to use this resource: the librarian there can help you get information that's intelligible to a layperson. Copy any materials that you want to study or share with your mate or his doctor, taking care to note the source (title, publisher, and date) on all materials. Remember, this is a stressful time in your life, and you may not be able to remember as much as you normally do!

Key Points about Doctor Visits

◊ Accompany the patient during all visits to the doctor so you can help gather information and provide support. If you are not able to accompany the patient, then someone who is close to the patient should.

◊ Familiarize yourself as soon as you can— preferably *before* visiting the doctor—with all possible testing procedures and treatment options.

◊ List any questions you have ahead of time, and take the list with you.

> ◊ Make notes and use a tape recorder during the visit. To help you make treatment decisions, you may want to take along a photocopy of the Stage-by-Stage Treatment Options chart that appears in this book (chapter 6), so that you can use it as a worksheet.
>
> ◊ Ask for copies of all medical records (such as test results) as they become available.

2. Talking with the Doctor about the Diagnosis.

As we've noticed in the recollections already presented, the final diagnosis can be communicated to the patient in a number of different ways, some of them more awkward and disturbing than others. It is not at all unusual for medical people to begin by speaking in jargon that the average patient can't immediately grasp, using expressions like *focal abnormality in the prostate*, or *Stage B/T2 growth*, or *adenocarcinoma*, or (as Allen heard) *positive 7*. According to Neil Shelton, a survivor of prostate cancer who researched the subject in 1993 for ABC television's *20/20* news program, the number one complaint expressed in prostate cancer support groups is that doctors don't communicate well with their patients; and in a 1991 survey of patients conducted by the American Medical Association, a startling 60 percent complained that their doctors didn't explain things in intelligible language.

Medical people who present the diagnosis in jargon are not being deliberately insensitive, although they certainly may be uncomfortable having to make this kind of unwelcome announcement. Rather, they are using the language that is the most familiar to them and that is the most "official," which, from their point of view, means it's the safest and the most authoritative. From the patient's point of view, however, this jargon can be extremely alienating.

It is also not unusual for patients to discover the diagnosis in a very offhand, and off-putting, manner, such as hearing it over the telephone from a nurse (as Leonard did). Many patients first learn their diagnosis by seeing it written on a report that they are told to carry from one place to another, or that is left open in front of them on an office table. As for the women whose lives will also be traumatized by the diagnosis, the news often gets communicated in the worst possible manner: by a loved one who is stricken with agony, completely dazed, or in full-blown denial.

If an ideal situation can be said to exist, it would be one in which the doctor meets with the patient *and* his partner and states clearly, "The tumor on your prostate is malignant." This situation is similar to what Tom and Rebecca experienced. However, in the ideal scenario, there would be an understanding *from the beginning of the diagnostic process* among the patient, his partner, and his doctor that every important discussion during that process would involve all of them meeting together. This approach, as opposed to the approach of not including the partner unless there's bad news, removes some of the anxiety from that final "announcement" meeting. It also helps to build more rapport among the principal players in the case, so that the doctor is likely to communicate the diagnosis more empathetically than Tom's doctor did to Tom and Rebecca.

In cases where the patient's partner is *not* the most appropriate person to accompany him during consultations with the doctor—for example, due to the partner's poor physical health or inability to cope with the emotional stress—then someone who is very close to the patient should be asked to do so (see chapter 5 for more information about building a personal support team). Throughout the rest of our discussion here, we'll assume that you, the partner, are accompanying the patient.

To better the chances of achieving the ideal consultation scenario, you and your partner might consider telling the doctor, at the very beginning of the diagnostic process, that, if at all possible, both of you want to be included in every major discussion pertaining to the case, and that both of you want important information communicated to you directly and privately by the doctor him- or herself. Also, whenever you or your partner are talking with the doctor—or any other medical authority—be sure to ask for an explanation of every term he or she uses that you do not understand.

After the announcement of the diagnosis comes the most challenging task in the doctor-patient-caregiver relationship, one that will be much easier if the steps mentioned above have been taken. Your partner and you need to resist the temptation to go limp: that is, to accept passively whatever the doctor says, or doesn't say, and remain "patient" in the most literal sense of the word. Instead, you need to keep the doctor engaged in a two-way dialogue, at the announcement meeting itself and at any subsequent meeting about the diagnosis, to make sure that every major issue gets addressed to everyone's satisfaction, and that all parties understand each other.

Here is where your role as a caregiver can be particularly effective. Your partner may be too preoccupied or disconcerted by his illness to make sure that all the right questions are being asked and answered, to keep track of what issues have, and have not, been adequately discussed, and to record all the information received in a thorough and efficient manner. Even more problematic, your partner may normally be what is known in the health-care world as an "avoider," someone who deliberately seeks to know as little as possible about a threatening experience in order to escape the stress of that knowledge. In either of these situations, you need to be what is known as a "vigilant": someone who seeks out as much relevant information as possible.

Presented below are twelve major questions that it is best to have your doctor answer as soon as possible after a diagnosis of prostate cancer:

1. What specific tests were conducted, and what were the specific results? How do these results compare with "normal"? What do these specific results mean? (NOTE: Aside from the *biopsy*, specific tests to ask about—i.e., that are commonly performed to obtain a diagnosis—include the *PSA test* and the *Gleason score*: see chapter 3)

2. How far advanced is the cancer—i.e., what *stage* has the cancer reached? (See chapter 2 for more information about staging.)

3. Are there other tests that might tell us more? What are they, and what is your opinion about their possible helpfulness?

4. How serious is this condition at the patient's age?

5. What is the full range of treatment options for this type of condition? (NOTE: See chapter 6 for a discussion of the major treatments for prostate cancer; this discussion—as well as any other background research you do—may prompt other questions for you to ask relating to specific options.)

6. For each of the treatment options that the doctor mentions, ask the following questions (also see the Stage-by-Stage Treatment Options chart in chapter 6):

   a. What is the likely outcome for a man of the patient's age, based on five-, seven-, and ten-year *follow-ups*?

   b. Assuming the doctor plans to administer the treatment him- or herself, how often does he or she normally do so in a month or a year? (NOTE: It should be relatively often, so that you can rely more confidently on his or her experience. If you're not sure whether the response means "often," check with another doctor or medical authority.)

   c. What is the typical process (or "treatment protocol") involved?

   d. How long does that process last? If hospitalization is involved, how long will that last? How long can the patient expect to be incapacitated and/or out of work?

   e. During and after the treatment, what kind of help will the patient need at home?

   f. What are the possible physical and emotional side effects? What can be done about these side effects?

    g. What is the cost range, and how much is likely to be covered by insurance?

7. Which treatment do you (the doctor) most recommend? Why? How would you rank the other treatments in terms of possible effectiveness for this patient? Why?

8. Would a *clinical trial* be appropriate for the patient? (NOTE: Clinical trials can take a number of forms. Usually, they involve a patient testing a new treatment that shows promise. In most cases, the patient not only has a chance of deriving unique benefits from such a treatment and of making a contribution to medical science, but also pays significantly less for treatment than he would in a nontrial context. In the treatment of prostate cancer, clinical trials are usually only available and recommended for advanced stages of the disease, when other alternatives seem inappropriate or ineffective.)

9. How quickly do we have to make a treatment decision? Why? (NOTE: In most cases, because prostate cancer is typically very slow to grow, there is time to do a substantial amount of your own research before having to make a final decision, and you should definitely take this time.)

10. In terms of the patient's present diet, activities, medications, and future plans, is there anything he should be doing—or should not be doing? Why?

11. Can you provide us with additional information, such as pamphlets, books, or videos? How can we find out more about this condition? (NOTE: Also see the "Resources" section in chapter 10 of this book. Tangible reference materials are especially valuable tools for helping family members and close friends to understand the illness.)

12. Can you recommend other doctors with whom to confer on this situation? (NOTE: Getting a "second opinion" for sure, and perhaps more opinions (depending on your— or the doctor's—uncertainty about the case), is universally considered advisable for any cancer diagnosis, and

will not offend the doctor. Indeed, it can help you, your partner, *and* the doctor to manage the illness more confidently. If the doctor does not seem to have much experience with a certain possible treatment option, it's especially important to speak with a doctor who does.)

Here are guidelines for conducting this type of doctor-patient-caregiver conversation more effectively:

◊ If possible, familiarize yourself with the diagnostic tests discussed in chapter 3 and the treatment options discussed in chapter 6. This will help you to comprehend and to speak the doctor's language.

◊ Prepare two copies of the list of questions you want to ask—one for your partner and one for you. Let your partner lead the conversation, because he is the one most affected by the illness; but be alert to initiate questions that your partner doesn't ask, or to ask for clarification when you don't understand something.

As a general rule, it's better not to give the doctor a written list of questions, or to ask the doctor for written replies to your questions. Face-to-face dialogue, in which you verbalize the questions and the doctor verbally responds, gives you and the doctor an opportunity to learn more about each other and to develop more rapport. However, if you normally have great difficulty conducting question-and-answer sessions of this type, you may want to let the doctor look at your list, or (if possible) send it to the doctor ahead of the meeting, if only to let him or her see the scope of the questions that you have.

◊ Try to avoid asking leading questions—ones that indirectly ask for a specific yes or no answer. For example, instead of saying, "I don't have to have surgery, do I?" which is certain to qualify your doctor's response, ask a more open-ended question like "What treatment options do you think apply to the situation?" Here are some other examples:

Leading Question	Open-Ended Question
Have you performed this procedure a lot?	How often have you performed this procedure over the past year? (With this question and others like it, consult some other medical authority if you're not sure how to interpret the quality of the answer)
How good is the nursing care in the hospital where he'll be going?	What training have the nurses had who will be caring for him in the hospital?
He's going to come out of this okay, isn't he?	What is the likely prognosis (or "outcome") for him?
Isn't it best to avoid surgery at all costs?	What do you feel about the possible pros and cons of surgery in this case?

You want the doctor's answers to be as honest and unbiased as possible, so that you can make the best possible decisions. For all their expertise in medical matters, doctors are not necessarily good at dialogue, and can, like anyone, fall into saying what they think their listeners *want* to hear, instead of what their listeners *need* to hear.

◊ Take copious notes during the conversation. If possible, bring a tape recorder with you and tape the conversation (a good idea for all future conversations as well). Research shows that people obtaining this kind of information frequently have stress-related trouble remembering it.

According to a 1992 study conducted at the Western General Hospital in Edinburgh, Scotland, cancer patients who had their consultations taped subsequently experienced lower levels of anxiety and remembered information concerning their illness, treatment options, and prognosis more effectively than patients who did not have their consultations taped. One of the caretakers interviewed for this book, a woman in her seventies who was with her husband when the doctor gave the diagnosis of advanced-stage prostate cancer, had this to report about the value of taping doctor-patient consultations:

> We didn't take a tape recorder into the doctor's office, and this became an issue between us—I heard one thing, and he heard another, and we argued about what the doctor had said. I was even angry at the doctor for not having told us to bring a tape recorder, which, of course, wasn't fair.

If you do tape-record your consultations, make sure to take written notes as well, in case the tape fails or gets lost. Also, have the doctor spell any unfamiliar terms so that you can investigate them later.

You should be aware that the doctor (like anyone else) may not be entirely comfortable with the idea of being tape-recorded. Some doctors may feel—consciously or subconsciously—that it represents a lack of trust on your part. Others may worry about the potential legal ramifications of the tape in the event that you wind up suing for malpractice. Because of these possibilities, it's best to explain in advance your need for, and right to make, a tape recording. and to ask for his or her cooperation.

It's wise to do as much as you can reasonably do to maintain a good doctor-patient-caregiver relationship, but first and foremost you must be sure to obtain the information that you need in order to understand what's going on. Tape recording can help give you this surety. After all, we're only human: when our ears hear something that they don't want to hear (like *cancer* or *surgery*), it's all too easy for them to stop listening.

- ◊ Try to visualize what's being explained to you. If you can't do so, ask the doctor for a picture or a demonstration.

- ◊ After receiving each piece of important information, repeat it to the doctor, to make sure that you've understood correctly.

- ◊ Always remember that no question is foolish under the circumstances, and that you have the right and the need to ask "Why?" "Why not?" "How?" "What?" and "When? "

◇   Don't put off asking the doctor for clarifications until "some other time"; instead, make sure that you understand matters *as you go along*. It's not only in your best interest to do this, it also benefits the doctor, whose schedule is usually very busy and highly subject to life-or-death crises. There's a natural limit to how often a doctor can repeat things—or tolerate repeating them, for that matter. The more effectively you work to understand and retain what your doctor says the first time you hear it, the less you will have to impose on him or her later.

◇   If you are having problems talking with, or understanding, the doctor, say so. If, during the course of the conversation, you feel overwhelmed, or underheard, tactfully bring this feeling to the doctor's attention. It can be very helpful to both of you!

◇   If you are unable to ask all the questions that you want to ask at the initial conference, schedule another, follow-up conference as soon as possible.

3. Determining if the Doctor is Right for the Patient.

In a situation as serious as a prostate cancer diagnosis, you and your partner don't want to take your doctor's expertise or compatibility for granted—nor would he or she expect you to do so! From both perspectives, there must be a good fit and an active two-way relationship between the patient-caretaker team and the physician. With this in mind, you and your partner need to do some checking and verifying so that you can answer yes to these questions knowledgeably and responsibly:

◇   Are you confident about your doctor's medical qualifications and recommendations?

◊ Are you satisfied with your doctor's hospital affiliation?

◊ Are you comfortable with your doctor's communication style?

Anatole Broyard, former editor of *The New York Times Book Review*, has written eloquently about the search for the right doctor. In the August 26, 1990, issue of *The New York Times Magazine*, he made a historically public and frank revelation of a prostate cancer diagnosis. He later incorporated this material in his 1992 book about battling prostate cancer, *Intoxicated by My Illness*. Here's a description of the kind of doctor that he said he was looking for in 1990 to supervise his future treatment:

> I would like a doctor who is not only a talented physician but a bit of a metaphysician, too, someone who can treat body and soul. I used to get restless when people talked about soul, but now I know better. Soul is the part of you that you summon up in emergencies. . . . To most physicians, my illness is a routine incident in their rounds, while for me, it's the crisis of my life. I would feel better if I had a doctor who at least perceived this incongruity.

Not every male patient may describe his ideal doctor in quite this way, but every male patient does need a doctor with whom he feels comfortable, safe, and supported: a doctor who not only displays medical expertise but also interacts well with his patient and his patient's caregiver(s) as individuals. This is all the more important in the case of a life-threatening illness like prostate cancer.

Some doctors, intentionally or unintentionally, may cause a prostate cancer patient to feel helpless, guilty, incompetent, or otherwise negative about himself, in which case the patient should definitely look for someone else. The doctor should be someone who inspires him—and you, his primary caretaker—to feel strength and hope, to be *re*moralized instead of *de*moralized.

First and foremost, however, your partner and you should be completely confident about the doctor's medical qualifications to handle the case. Here are the issues to check, through direct communication with the doctor, and through research with the doctor's staff or hospital administration:

⬥ What is the doctor's educational background and training?

⬥ How long has the doctor practiced in his or her current capacity?

⬥ With what hospital, organizations, and institutions is the doctor professionally affiliated?

⬥ What kind of services can this doctor and this hospital provide?

⬥ What are the doctor's special areas of expertise?

⬥ How extensive is the doctor's experience with prostate cancer patients of the same age?

In addition, many patients and their caregivers find it beneficial to talk with anyone they know who has been, or is, a patient of this doctor's. Such conversations can offer unique insights into what an experience with that doctor might be like, from both a medical and interpersonal perspective. If you don't know any other patients personally, try asking around among your relatives, friends, and support group members.

Finally, you and your partner should mentally assess every encounter that you have with the doctor in terms of its "comfort level," given the circumstances. Each of you should be able to answer yes to all of the following questions—not only during the initial interview with the doctor but also throughout the course of your relationship with the doctor:

⬥ Does the doctor explain everything well?

⬥ Bearing in mind that the doctor may not be able to give definitive answers to some of your questions, does the doctor answer all of your questions clearly, promptly, thoughtfully, and (to the best of your knowledge) competently?

⬧ Does the interaction you have with the doctor seem like a dialogue rather than a monologue on the doctor's part?

⬧ Does the doctor take into account *your* concerns, opinions, and preferences as well as his or her own?

⬧ Does the doctor take care to make sure that you understand what he or she is saying?

⬧ Does the doctor seem genuinely interested in the patient and the particular nature of the patient's illness?

⬧ Does the doctor allow sufficient time for the visit, and does the doctor give his or her full attention to your partner and you during this time?

⬧ Do you leave the doctor's company feeling reasonably clear and confident about the next phase of the case?

Whether or not your partner and you are content with the doctor who has given the diagnosis, you should definitely seek a second opinion before making any treatment-related decisions. If nothing else, it will serve to validate what your doctor has already told you. You should also conduct your own research into prostate cancer, so that you will be better equipped to make judgments based on what your doctor says (see the section "Resources" in chapter 10).

4. Informing Others about the Diagnosis.

People have different emotional responses and timetables. Some men diagnosed with prostate cancer instinctively want to hide the news as much as possible from the people around them. Other men instinctively want to reach out to people by sharing the news. Some men are emotionally ready to talk with people about their diagnosis immediately afterward. Other men require more time to adjust to the diagnosis before they're ready for such talks.

Since family members, friends, and close business associates are almost certain to learn about the diagnosis sooner or later, it might be best for your partner (or someone speaking on his behalf, like you) to discuss the diagnosis with these people as soon as possible. This approach enables people who care very much about the patient to offer valuable love and support right from the start—something that helps them, as well as the patient *and* his caregiver, to cope more effectively with the illness and its consequences.

In some cases, the patient's diagnosis might have a direct bearing on other people's future plans, adding an extra dimension to the need for timely disclosure. Adult children, for example, may want as much advance notice as they can get in order to avoid having to be away during a patient's critical operation; or an employer may need to know as much as he or she can in order to start rearranging workloads to accommodate a possibly lengthy convalescence.

What's best, however, is not always obtainable. People in the patient's life, especially those nearest to him, need to respect the fact that it is his right to tell others about his illness when and how he wishes. As the primary caregiver, you can and should help him to do what's best, but you shouldn't force him. Here are some guidelines:

- ◊ No one should be told without your partner's knowledge and permission. Ideally, your partner should do the telling, because that in itself creates a special bond between your partner and the person being told. It's okay, however, for someone else to do the telling if the partner prefers. The designated teller should inform the person being told that your partner specifically requested the telling.

- ◊ Whenever the news is told to someone, sufficient time should be allowed for the informed person to respond however he or she wishes and for all questions to be answered. The best time to tell someone is when both parties have at least an hour that's free from distractions.

◊ The teller should be as open and honest as he or she can be in expressing the news. False cheer is definitely not appropriate. Sincere optimism is.

◊ Your partner or his designated teller should be prepared to offer written materials about prostate cancer to the person being told, so that he or she can better understand the illness. It's generally better not to mention or give out these materials until *after* there's been sufficient time to talk, or the materials may be distracting. The best course of action may be to give or send them to the person at a later time.

◊ The teller should be prepared for the fact that the news may trigger unexpected and/or unwanted feelings in the person being told. For example, the person may react with an outpouring of affection that is uncharacteristic and, to some degree, embarrassing; or the person may be disconcertingly emotionless; or the person may burst out with anger, perhaps even anger directed against the teller. Whatever the case, special consideration and acceptance is warranted. The person being told shouldn't be held to account for the way he or she behaves at that particular time, given the especially stressful nature of the communication.

◊ Don't avoid telling a child on the grounds that he or she is too young to understand or accept the news. The child is almost certain to sense that something is going on, and may easily imagine that the situation is worse than it is. Just make sure to accommodate the child's age and maturity level. For example, a patient might start telling the news to a seven-year-old grandchild in this manner:

> The doctors tell me that I'm very sick, but they're pretty sure they can make me well. It's

not a sickness like a cold or chicken pox. It's very different. It is not a sickness you can catch. Sometimes I may not be feeling good, and sometimes I may be sad or grouchy. I just want you to know that it's nothing you've done, and that I need you to be patient and understanding. Will you please do this for me?

Always give the child ample opportunity to express his or her feelings and to ask questions. However, don't be surprised if the child says very little. This is quite normal, and the child shouldn't be pressured to react if no reaction is immediately forthcoming. And remember, someone else can break the news to a child if your partner or you are uncomfortable doing so.

◊ Your partner may need considerable time sorting out his feelings of anger, fear, or inner confusion before he is ready to talk with other people about the illness, even though other people may already know that he's been diagnosed as having it. In this case, your partner (or you) should try to postpone any conversation by saying, "I appreciate your concern but I (he) just can't talk about it right now." In the next chapter, you and your partner will find ways of coping with common emotional difficulties and communication problems involved in coping with a prostate cancer diagnosis.

5

Dealing with the Diagnosis: Emotional Issues

⬥ How patients react emotionally to a diagnosis

⬥ How caregivers react emotionally to a diagnosis

⬥ How to set up an effective support system among family members and friends

⬥ Coping strategies: improving caregiver-partner communication, keeping a journal, breathing for relaxation

Any man who receives the diagnosis "cancer," and any woman who hears that her partner has received this diagnosis, will react as if the entire world has suddenly changed. And it has.

As a caregiver, you know this, and so does the man for whom you care. Gone is the personal shield of invulnerability that each of you had naively assumed would protect you forever. All at once, you are face to face with ugly realities that the shield once obscured—including the most unsettling fact of all: that bad things like major illness and death do not just happen to other people, they happen to you as well. Whatever the final outcome of your encounter with cancer, your life will never be the same again.

In this chapter, we will explore how this upsetting new world can initially feel, both to the patient and to you, the caregiver. Then we will discuss ways to cope with these feelings, so that both of you—as well as the family and friends who support you—can get through the crisis of prostate cancer as effectively as possible, gaining new insights and skills to enhance the new life before you. We'll begin by focusing on the patient's emotional responses.

The Patient's Emotional Responses

As we discussed in chapters 1 and 4, a man with prostate cancer generally has a variety of emotional responses to the illness, many of which may not be observable to an outsider. Each man's repertoire of responses is based on a number of factors: his overall psychological character; his prior experience with illness and trauma (although a man diagnosed with prostate cancer may not actually *feel* sick); his attitudes toward aging, sex, and masculinity; and his concept of what *cancer* means.

In the time immediately after the diagnosis, your partner's emotional responses can shift dramatically and unpredictably from hour to hour, day to day, and week to week, adding to his stress and, directly or indirectly, to the stress of those around him. As his caretaker, you need to accept that this emotional shifting is bound to occur.

In addition to accepting this fact, you may find it helpful to keep reminding yourself that no two people are the same: your partner may not feel or behave quite like any other man, nor may he feel or behave quite like you. Most important, this difference in feeling or behaving doesn't mean your partner is "wrong." In any life situation, but especially in a crisis situation, we need to respect our differences just as we relish our similarities.

The more carefully—and considerately—you are able to identify and track your partner's emotional responses to his diagnosis, the better equipped you will be to help him and yourself to cope with these responses. This does *not* mean that you have to "fix" your partner's emotional responses. Playing "psychologist" at home is an unrealistic burden to impose on yourself, and it is very likely to backfire. Aside from making your mate feel uncomfortable and even hostile, which can only aggravate any preexisting problems in your relationship, your efforts to "fix" his emotional reactions might actually intensify them. He may come to think, for example, that expressing these emotions is a justifiable means of declaring his personal rights and needs as distinguished from your particular rights and needs.

Instead of *fixing* your partner's responses, however negative they may appear, try to focus on *understanding* his responses, so that you can do whatever you reasonably can to ensure that they upset him—and you—as little as possible. Later in this chapter, we'll have more specific suggestions on how to cope with a partner's negative feelings when they prove too upsetting. For now, let's simply look more closely at what these feelings may be.

Discussed below are some of the most common emotional reactions experienced by men who have just been diagnosed with prostate cancer. These issues are not presented in any particular order, and they overlap in many cases. In reviewing them, bear in mind that your goal is not to "label" your partner in terms of a particular type of emotional response pattern but, rather, to develop more sensitivity toward a variety of responses that can come and go in the life of *any* man during this crisis penod.

◊ *Denial and disbelief*: The patient avoids facing the diagnosis itself by focusing attention on some other issue. This reaction is often characterized by "avoidance" statements like "This can't be happening to me" or "It's no big deal"; by "hypothetical" statements like "If only I had been tested earlier"; or by "undoing" statements like "Please make it yesterday." It's also characterized by sensations of things being "unreal."

◊ *Anger:* The patient, feeling threatened and outraged, expresses hostility toward the doctor, himself, his partner, or even the world in general. He feels he's been victimized ("Why me?") and is looking for a fight.

◊ *Fear:* The patient's anxiety is translated into displays of terror or panic, or rash statements like "I just want to get the cancer cut out of me as quickly as possible."

◊ *Depression:* Overwhelmed by the diagnosis, the patient feels a physical and emotional exhaustion that makes him listless. Along with this listlessness can come feelings of hopelessness and defeat.

In everyday speech, the word *depression* is commonly used to mean the same thing as *sadness*, which is how it is used here as well. Psychologically speaking, however, the word *depression* refers to a more severe, complicated, and long-term illness, which in some cases can provoke suicidal thoughts or activities. Fortunately, clinical depression (as the illness is called) can often be overcome by specific medical and/or psychological treatment. For a description of clinical depression and a discussion of suicidal indicators, see the section "Emotional Issues" in chapter 8. In the meantime, if your partner does engage in suicidal thoughts or activities at any time, you should immediately consult with your doctor or, if your doctor is not immediately available, with your local hospital emergency room. It's never worth taking a chance!

◊ *Loss of control:* The patient is preoccupied with the fact that the illness is upsetting his life and his plans. It renders him passive and bewildered. He may exhibit uncharacteristic carelessness, thoughtlessness, or incompetence.

◊ *Desire to control:* Feeling helpless and/or belittled in the face of the diagnosis, the patient tries to exercise as much control over other aspects of his life as he can. He may also do everything he can to control the treatment process for his illness ("Order me books: I have to get to the bottom of this!"). This "complete control" goal can be therapeutic to a certain degree, but it can also create unnecessary and counterproductive problems in his interactions with doctors and caregivers.

◊ *Need for isolation:* The patient feels very self-conscious with all this sudden attention to his vulnerability and seeks to be alone.

◊ *Silence:* Given the potentially calamitous implications of the diagnosis, the patient either doesn't know what to say, or fears saying something wrong, or associates silence with strength (the macho ideal of the "strong, silent type"). Often the silence-response is motivated by a desire not to worry others, especially his partner.

◊ *Mourning:* The patient feels devastated by the diagnosis, and experiences a deep sense of loss. It may be characterized by statements like "My life will never be the same again" or "It was the end of the world for me." A mourning response may also prompt the patient to dwell on all the things that he has not accomplished in his life.

◊ *Flight:* The patient literally runs around doing things that will keep him from having to deal with the diagnosis. Often a "flight" reaction, the counterpart of a "fight" or "anger" reaction, involves getting away from the home—the personal world that he considers most affected (or "infected") by the diagnosis. Typically, a patient's flight is toward escapist activities: e.g., reading, sports, movies, gambling, drinking; but it may also be toward increased involvement in his work.

⬦   *Guilt and shame:* Any illness can make a patient feel
     as if he or she is somehow flawed, or has somehow
     failed. A cancer diagnosis, however, carries its own
     special stigma. In popular culture, the development
     of cancer in a person is often attributed to harboring
     (or repressing) negative character traits, such as hos-
     tility, depression, anxiety, or grief; or to being some-
     how blocked in one's emotional or spiritual
     development Given such a cultural bias, a man may
     respond to a diagnosis of prostate cancer by doubt-
     ing, blaming, or criticizing himself.

     In fact, there is not yet any scientific basis for
     the notion of a "cancer-prone personality"—a
     notion inspired by the fact that cancer's causes are
     so mysterious and by the human need to have some
     control over that mystery. In other words, we have
     no proof that one's personal character and attitude
     can play a deciding role in keeping cancer at bay.

     We do know that stress can aggravate *any*
     chronic illness. If you suffer from chronic back pain,
     you know that your back becomes an indicator of
     your stress level; if you suffer from chronic colitis,
     it's your intestines; if you suffer from chronic
     asthma, its your lungs. You can't consciously con-
     trol this situation. Nevertheless, a person's mind *can*
     serve as a powerful healer during the course of any
     illness, helping him or her to withstand pain, to
     cope more effectively with treatment, and to adjust
     to the long-range consequences of illness. Always
     bear in mind that *healing* a person (literally, making
     that person "whole") is a different process from *cur-
     ing* his or her illness.

Most caregivers find that the best way of dealing with any or
all of these emotional reactions is, first of all, to be as tolerant,
understanding, and tactful as they reasonably can. For a while at
least, try to avoid confrontations or dramatic actions aimed at
"jolting" your partner out of his mood. He may need time to
adjust to the diagnosis on his own terms as best he can.

Meanwhile, it may be helpful for you to take note of *when* such reactions occur, *what form* they take, and *how long* they last. If you can identify certain situations that tend to trigger, aggravate, or prolong troublesome reactions, you may be able to do something about those situations: either prevent them from happening or alter their character so that they don't have as strong an effect. For example, you may not want to schedule social engagements if you find that they upset your partner emotionally. You may want to postpone undertaking new projects at home if you sense that they may intensify your partner's feelings of helplessness and incompetence. You may want to make breakfast time more special if you've noticed that your partner's depression is most acute during the early morning hours.

Your Emotional Responses as a Caretaker

At the same time that you are monitoring your partner's emotional reactions, you should also be monitoring your own. Partners of people with serious illnesses can experience the same types of emotional reactions we've already examined, as well as the following reactions:

- ◊ *Emotional isolation:* Accustomed to sharing emotions with the patient, the partner now feels as if she's left all alone with her feelings, which can translate into anxiety and despair.

- ◊ *Resentment:* The partner is overwhelmed not only by the diagnosis, but also by the prospect (or actuality) of "role reversal," i.e., having to take on some of the functions that the patient has previously handled: for example, managing the family budget, driving at night, or engaging outside help for repair and maintenance tasks (all tasks that the man typically manages in a "traditional" marriage). She might be especially likely to feel resentment if the patient has never shared his experience in handling such functions, thus leaving her completely unprepared to take them over. Her resentment over these matters can become even stronger if the patient is simultaneously acting cold or antagonistic toward her.

◊ *Engulfment:* The partner is so absorbed by the patient's needs that she loses sense of her own independent identity and needs (the so-called "selflessness trap"). The result is a loss of energy—physical and emotional—and, possibly, depression.

◊ *Entitlement:* Faced with the prospect (or actuality) of a dramatic change in her day-to-day life, the partner feels that she will lose, or is losing, something that she deserves, through no fault of her own. As a result, she may feel indignant toward the patient, her family members, and her friends for not giving her "compensatory" attention (in many cases, an unrealistic expectation on her part) and self-righteous toward the world in general for being unfair and uncaring.

◊ *Escapist fantasies:* The partner may be unable to resist wishing that she could be released from her present situation of uncertainty and emotional turmoil (sometimes coupled with physical exhaustion). For example, she may find herself repeatedly imagining a life apart from the patient, either alone or with another man. This is a particularly natural response if the partner is unaccustomed to feeling pity for the patient, or to thinking of him as vulnerable, and isn't sure how to deal with such feelings and thoughts. The partner may even develop fantasies about the patient's death, if only to test out what her reaction might be. These are very common and perfectly normal responses.

Although it may be difficult for you to think about caring for yourself at a time like this, when your partner's life may be at stake, it is vital that you do so—for his good as well as for your own. The best way to begin coping with any of the emotions that have just been described is to be tolerant toward yourself. If possible, try to change or avoid situations that seem especially likely to spark or intensify such reactions. And seek the emotional support of a good friend: someone with whom you have a strong, independent relationship and who has proved to be loyal and empathetic in the past.

Later in this chapter, we'll look at how you can communicate more effectively with your partner, after the diagnosis, about specific emotional issues that may be affecting your relationship. First, however, let's look at a coping component that can mean a great deal both to your partner and to yourself: a well-organized support system of family members and friends.

Creating an Effective Support System

In coping with any serious illness, it's best for the patient and his caregiver to start creating a support system immediately after the diagnosis, before the demands of the illness or the treatment consume too much of their time and energy. A support system is a network of people apart from the medical team itself who may sooner or later be able to provide practical assistance and/or emotional succor to the patient or the caretaker. The earlier the members of this support team are recruited and brought into the information pipeline, the better equipped they are to help when help is needed.

Work with your partner to identify in advance people who might be helpful to either or both of you during the course of the illness and any treatment associated with the illness. These people include:

◊ One particularly close and trustworthy relative or friend who can be the "second-in-command" caretaker: someone to take over matters (such as keeping everyone else informed) if you are too busy.

◊ Friends and relatives who can serve as possible chauffeurs, shoppers, house-sitters, or "convalescence aides."

◊ Friends and relatives who can be counted on to provide emotional comfort and support, to your partner and/or you, when it's needed.

Keep in mind that just being *surrounded* by people, no matter how well intentioned they may be, does not constitute being *supported*. True support is having access to the particular quality of a relationship that you need at a given time. This means, for example, that if what you urgently need is information, then having a loving person around who does not possess that information will not be supportive for you. Likewise, if what you need is an understanding, empathetic person, then the most well-informed family member or friend will not be supportive if he or she is incapable of empathic understanding.

One way of addressing this issue, developed by Dr. Barbara, is to think in terms of a tri-level model of support. This model divides a well-functioning support system into three essential levels:

Level 1 = casual support
Level 2 = functional support
Level 3 = intimate support

Let's consider each level separately:

Level 1: The people who fit into this category are acquaintances. They are people whom you acknowledge—and who acknowledge you—in a relatively superficial way. To a limited degree, you share common experiences with them, and you offer each other mutual aid. A "Level 1" person might be someone you meet at a bus stop or in a grocery store, a nurse on a single shift of your hospital stay, or the receptionist in your doctor's office.

These are your typical "Have a nice day!" people who may, in fact, be able to offer you special services just when they're needed: a drive to the hospital, a home-service reference, or simply a kind word and open ear. If you think that it's not important to maintain these relationships in your life, particularly when you or your loved one is feeling ill and powerless, try going through an entire day without anyone acknowledging your existence.

Level 2: People who fit into this category are people with whom you've developed an ongoing relationship that isn't deeply personal, but that does have some substance to it. "Level 2" people might include your regular tennis partner, a colleague at work or a member of a patient support group: someone who regularly cooperates with you in projects, provides information or services, shares in your activities, or makes you feel part of a group. These are people upon whom you can count for companionship, simple tasks, and thoughtful concern. You may never expose any of your innermost feelings to a "Level 2" person, but you can recruit them from time to time to play functional roles on your support team.

Level 3: The people who fit into this category are the ones who are truly special to you, particularly now that you face the hardships of a life-threatening illness. These are your true intimates, the ones with whom you can let down your hair, and with whom you can share your most personal self. "Level 3" people can be counted on to help you with the most logistically difficult and emotionally distressing parts of the illness experience.

In many cases, one person in a couple has more "Level 3" people in his or her life—or is more accustomed to developing such relationships—than the other. Typically, this person is the woman, since women are culturally more conditioned to seek intimacy. But *both* partners need people—other than each other—who can offer personal "Level 3" support. In situations where no "Level 3" support is available to a particular individual, it may be wise to seek someone from the helping professions (for example, a psychologist or social worker)—a person who is qualified to deal responsibly and effectively with health crises and emotional issues in general. In fact, even when "Level 3" people are available to you, you may find significant benefit from seeking the help of a psychotherapist.

You might try listing the people in your own life, in your partner's life, and in your life as a couple who fit into each of these categories. Then, if you find that a particular category seems rather empty, you would be wise to work on filling it: for example, by establishing better relationships with casual acquaintances or friends. As soon as you have identified people who might fulfill different tasks or levels of support on your support team, you and your partner should both start trying to recruit them. Whenever you can, let them know what you might be—and might not be—needing from them in the near future. In some cases, you can have this discussion at the same time as you announce the diagnosis. In other cases, you may want to wait until you've seen how individual people react to the diagnosis, or until you've made a specific treatment decision.

In addition to talking with family members and friends about being available for support, you and your partner should also consider doing the following:

◊   Join a local support group for cancer patients in general, and/or prostate cancer patients specifically, and their partners. Ask your doctor, and see the "Resources" section in chapter 10 of this book.

◊   Investigate the resources that exist to meet your spiritual needs. At a time of crisis in your life, these needs are bound to become more intense. Some people already have ties with spiritual groups or religious institutions, in which case they can work to strengthen these ties. Other people follow a more personal path, in which case they should make sure to allow themselves the time and the means for doing spiritual work throughout the illness experience, and they should strengthen contacts with others who have similar beliefs.

Improving Communication

A time of crisis, like confronting a diagnosis of prostate cancer, makes good communication between a person and his partner essential to the couple's emotional survival. Unfortunately, it also makes good communication much harder to achieve. Crises tend to aggravate the core communication problems that two people develop over the course of their relationship, but are able to over-look or even to forget during less critical times.

In addition, crises tend to make people much more concerned about issues of "tone" in a conversation—i.e., whether the words they're hearing sound sympathetic or cold, genuine or sarcastic, supportive or threatening. Ironically, at the same time that people are experiencing this heightened concern about the tone of a conversation, they're also becoming more predisposed to misinterpret that tone, based on their own deepening fears and sensitivities.

To make matters potentially even more complicated, there are common, culturally conditioned differences between the way men communicate and the way women communicate (for more on this subject, see chapter 1). In a male-female relationship, these differences, which can be intriguing in happier times, can easily become exasperating during a crisis.

In the emotionally disconcerting period following a diagnosis of prostate cancer in particular, male-female couples typically experience one or more of three major communication difficulties:

1. Conversation on the topic provokes anger, hurt, resentment, frustration, or other strong negative reactions.

2. Conversation on the topic seems superficial, false, indirect, or otherwise unsatisfying.

3. The patient does not—and perhaps will not—talk about the topic at all.

Let's consider each of these problems separately.

1. Conversation on the Topic Provokes Anger, Hurt, Resentment, Frustration, or other Strong Negative Emotions.

In any discussion of a sensitive issue, it is easy for a dialogue to degenerate into a parallel monologue: each person preoccupied with what he or she has to say and listening only passively—or reactively—to the other person. Thus we have the following kinds of potentially troublesome exchanges:

Dialogue A

He: "I'm not sure I want to go to another doctor just yet."

She: "But your life is at stake here. You have to go, and the sooner the better."

Likely Outcome: Either one person gives up out of frustration, thereby feeling resentful, or both people refuse to budge from their points of view, resulting in both people feeling angry.

Dialogue B

He: "This is something I can manage by myself. There's no need for you to get all upset."

She: "Okay, I was just trying to help."

Likely Outcome: She will wind up feeling unappreciated, rejected, and possibly indignant at his assumption that she would just "get all upset." He will wind up feeling alternately pressured by her concern and guilty for dismissing it.

Dialogue C

He: "I can't sleep at night. I can't get anything done during the day. It seems like my whole life is falling apart! "

She: "Well, maybe you should just take a break for a while. Clear your schedule and don't worry about getting anything done."

Likely Outcome: He will remain too agitated to simply accept her advice—which may, in fact, not meet his needs—and, as a result, he will feel alienated from her, even annoyed by her calmness. She, on the other hand, despite her compassion, will feel ignored and possibly a bit contemptuous of his refusal to see the wisdom of her advice.

What's needed to improve the likely outcome of each dialogue is active listening. Essentially, active listening is a four-step process:

1. Withholding any reactions for a while;

2. paying complete attention to what the other person is saying;

3. letting the other person know that you are listening by reflecting what he or she says; and

4. helping that person to express himself or herself as accurately and completely as possible before finally responding with your feelings and thoughts (should you choose—or need—to do so).

In each of the above dialogues, both people remain focused on their own personal point of view. The woman *reacts* to what she hears, but she doesn't *act* upon what she hears. Instead, she activates her own feelings or thoughts. Let's examine how each dialogue could be improved by active listening:

Dialogue A

He: "I'm not sure I want to go to another doctor just yet."

She: "So, you'd rather wait for a while before going to see another doctor." (She reflects what she's heard by virtually repeating it; and because he feels heard, he's more inclined to open up.)

He: "That's right. I'd like to do some research on my own first so that I know what to ask." (By being given a chance to explain himself more fully, he expresses a rationale that makes her less likely to panic).

Dialogue B

He: "This is something I can manage by myself. There's no need for you to get upset."

She: "I see; what you're saying is that you don't want me to worry." (She reflects his language without insinuating any meaning into it.)

He: "Well, I realize that I can't keep you from worrying to a certain extent, but I have a plan that I think will work out for this."

She: "You have a plan." (She reflects his words to get him to say more—a subtler, less threatening approach than a direct question, although a tactful direct question would be a final resort.)

He: "Yes, let me tell you about it." (The sharing of the plan helps bring the two people together. In going over the plan with her, he may even think of a way that she *can* help).

Dialogue C

He: "I can't sleep at night. I can't get anything done during the day. It seems like my whole life is falling apart! "

She: "That's awful. I imagine you feel pretty helpless." (She reflects that she has heard him by empathizing with him, and she invites him to clarify his feelings by sharing how she has heard him.)

He: "Well, it's more like being overwhelmed. I really need to get better organized and maybe enlist one or two people to take over some of my work." (By being assisted to think more deeply about his feelings, he comes up with a viable solution.)

Ideally, both the patient and the caregiver will practice active listening whenever it's necessary. However, one person practicing it is a good start—and a good example!

2. Conversation on the Topic Seems Superficial, False, Indirect, or Otherwise Unsatisfying.

As we've seen in the previous section, active listening can help to sustain, deepen, direct, and illuminate conversations so that they are far more satisfying. Taking the time and energy to reflect the patient's language, thoughts, and feelings not only demonstrates to him in the best possible way that you're interested in what he has to say, but also makes him more interested in talking with you.

However, there are two other factors to consider if your conversations tend to be shallow, sketchy, or off-hand:

◇ Do you pick the right time and place to talk? It should be a time when you are relatively relaxed and can devote yourself to the conversation, and it should be a place where you won't be distracted or uncomfortable.

◇ Do you keep the conversation focused on the topic, instead of allowing the conversation to meander as it will? Although sometimes the two of you may refer to the topic very briefly in the course of a more general conversation, there should also be times when a whole conversation—or a lengthy stretch of conversation—is devoted solely to the topic.

Let's look at an instructive example of how a potentially serious discussion about a troubling test result can be sabotaged and rendered superficial, false, or indirect. A family is seated around the dinner table—Father, Mother, Susy, and George:

Susy starts telling a story about a friend. Father, clearly preoccupied, turns away from Susy, fidgets, and finally says to Mother, "Remind me to tell you what happened at my appointment today."

Mother, feeling obliged to respond to Father, says, "How did it go?" Susy stops talking, but radiates frustration at being interrupted, which is apparent to everyone else at the table and undercuts the rest of the conversation.

Father then says, "Well, the appointment was very interesting. His office is in the Medical Arts Building."

George interjects, "Oh, I know that building. My friend has an office there too. It's nice. Did you notice the new sculpture out front?" This is what's known as "tangential" communication: George is chattering away to relieve his anxiety about what Father may be about to reveal. Father, meanwhile, is frustrated—and put off his intended tone—by the interruption.

Mother resumes the conversation: "What did the doctor say?"

Father answers, "The blood tests are questionable."

Mother says, "What did he mean, they're questionable?"

Father says, "I don't really know, but I'm sure it's okay."

Mother says, "If it's okay, why didn't the doctor call the house instead of having you come in?" With this remark, Mother is using the power of the questioner to take the floor away from Father. Questions can be benign, helpful allies, if they lead to where the speaker wants or needs to go. But they can be counterproductive if they relate only to the questioner's issues.

Father responds, "How should I know? Anyway, everything's okay so far, so until we hear more, let's just drop the matter."

The above conversation is unsatisfactory because it is poorly timed and too open to interruption. In a more private conversation between Father and Mother, devoted solely to the topic of the visit to the doctor, active listening skills would be easier to practice. Thus, the following, more productive exchange, for example, could occur:

Father: "The doctor said the blood tests are questionable."

Mother: "The blood tests are questionable. . . . How do you feel about that?"

Father: "Well, it's a bit uncomfortable."

Mother: "Uncomfortable, yes, and it sounds scary too."

Father: "Yes, it does, I guess, but we can deal with it if we go one step at a time. Why don't you come with me to my next appointment?" (Encouraged by her understanding, he does wind up saying what was in the back of his mind all along.)

3. The Patient Does Not—and Perhaps Will Not—Talk about the Topic at All.

Again, active listening can go far to make the patient want to talk, but you can't begin listening until he starts talking. While it's important to respect the patient's right to deal with the diagnosis in his own way, it's also important to make sure that you and the patient understand each other's feelings and needs. Too much silence can make this understanding impossible.

Initially, you can try the following, very tolerant ways of dealing with your partner's tendency to lapse into silence for extended periods of time:

◊ Before "silence attacks" occur, discuss what would be helpful to each of you. For example, your partner may feel that it would help him to get over his "silent attacks" earlier and more easily if you were indulgent and affectionate (perhaps giving him a hug from time to time) while they lasted. You, on the other hand, may feel the need for your partner to say something very simple, but specific, that will give you hope, such as "I just don't feel like talking now. How about right before dinner?"

◊ Agree to a "time-out" period: i.e., that it will be okay to have some mutual silence for a while. Depending on the situation, it might be a good idea to set a deadline for this period, a time when you can look forward to talking.

◊   You, the caretaker, can write your questions, con-
    cerns, and feelings in a letter to your partner. Then,
    give this letter to your partner and tell him to read it
    when he wants to, and to arrange a good time to
    discuss it with you when he's ready.

For some couples, the need to communicate about certain
issues may be more pressing, in which case you can try some of
the following strategies.

Many patients wait for their partners to take the lead in a
conversation about sensitive, illness-related issues, but their partners avoid doing so, either because they don't know what to say
or they don't want to put the patient on the spot. If this sounds
like your situation, remember that even a clumsy conversation
opener is usually better than silence. Try asking, "Please tell me a
little about what you're feeling today" or some open-ended
question—one that can't be dismissed with a simple yes or no.

In some cases, a patient actively discourages any conversation, claiming that it's the only way he can cope with the diagnosis (an "avoidance" or "denial" reaction). When faced with this
type of stonewalling, try expressing gently, in a nonaccusatory
manner, your need to talk, and be prepared to keep the conversation going by stating your feelings, concerns, and questions (Thus
giving him an opportunity to try some active listening!).

Another way to overcome silence on this topic is for you and
your partner to communicate with each other directly and immediately in writing, a method used in "Marriage Encounter" work-
shops that's proven effective for couples faced with many
different kinds of personal and interpersonal crises. First, you and
your partner agree on a subject to discuss, and then, independently, you write about that subject for several minutes. The writing time should be relatively brief, since you simply want to jot
down the major thoughts or feelings that first come to mind. Sample sentences that you may want to use as starting points are:

◊   When I first heard the diagnosis, I felt . . .

◊   What I fear most about the diagnosis is . . .

◊   What I need most from you at this time is . . .

After you've each written your responses, you exchange them, so that each of you can read what the other has written. The two of you are then free to discuss, or not to discuss, the writings: either way, you have shared something important with each other.

If your partner remains uncommunicative despite all these strategies, avoid lapsing into silence yourself. Keep letting him know, indirectly, that you're receptive to conversation whenever he's ready by regularly conveying your love, interest, and support. Above all, try not to complain, nag, or goad him into speaking. This will only make him defensive and therefore unlikely to share his deepest, most sensitive feelings with you.

Throughout the rest of this book, we'll talk about different ways that you can communicate more effectively with your partner during the course of the illness and afterward. Now let's look at two coping activities that can help you *or* him privately manage any distressing emotional responses to the illness, beginning with your reactions to the diagnosis: keeping a journal and breathing for relaxation.

Keeping a Journal

One of the most effective ways to identify, track, and process day-to-day emotions is to keep a daily journal about them. This activity is particularly helpful for men. Repeated studies have shown that men typically find it much more difficult than women to identify and describe their feelings in words. Scientists label this difficulty "alexithymia," and psychologist Dr. Ronald Levant, formerly of the Harvard Medical School, attributes its prevalence among men to social conditioning:

> Not only were boys not encouraged to identify and express their emotions, but more pointedly they were told not to. They might have been told that "big boys don't cry," and admonished to learn to "play with pain." These exhortations trained them to be out of touch with their feelings, particularly those feelings on the vulnerable end of the spectrum. As a result of such

socialization experiences, men are often genuinely unaware of their emotions. Lacking this emotional awareness, they tend to rely on cognition and try to logically deduce how they should feel. They cannot do what is automatic for most women—simply sense inward, feel the feeling, and let the verbal description come to mind.

Fortunately, men *can* learn to be more in touch with their feelings, and journal keeping (essentially a cognitive activity) is an excellent learning tool for this purpose. Remember, also, that some men are very verbal in general, but simply never learned to be verbal about their personal emotions in particular.

Consider, for example, American writer Cornelius Ryan, author of popular World War II histories like *The Longest Day* (1959) and *A Bridge Too Far* (1974). When Ryan discovered that he had prostate cancer in 1974, he started keeping a journal of the experience. "It served a therapeutic use," he said. "To record unsettling thoughts and feelings in the journal, away from the presence of others, eased the awful feeling that I was under a sentence of death."

Ryan's journal eventually became *A Private Battle*, the 1979 best-selling account of his fight with prostate cancer; but this didn't happen until after he died, and his wife, discovering the journal, added her own commentary to it about her wrenching experiences as his caretaker. *A Private Battle* remains a moving and instructive account of how a patient and his caretaker coped with prostate cancer, although current readers must bear in mind that major advances in prostate cancer diagnosis, treatment, and "consciousness" have been made since the book was written.

Here are some tips for recording one's emotional life in a journal, whether one is a patient or a caretaker:

◊   Describe the circumstances surrounding each major emotion—pleasurable and painful—that you felt during the day: the sequence of events that preceded it, the time and place of occurrence, how and why it seemed to pass. These details can provide clues for increasing the future incidence of pleasurable feelings and decreasing the future incidence of painful feelings. (NOTE: See the following page for a list of common emotions.)

 ⬥ Make a concerted effort to identify and describe the *physical* feelings that accompanied the *emotional* feelings, so that you can begin to make connections between the two. Anger, for example, might manifest itself physically as a sensation of heat, a clenching of the muscles, a quickening of the heartbeat, and/or an upset stomach. Fear may be most often experienced when one is tired, hungry, or uncomfortably chilly. The more sensitive you are to such connections, the more control you have over them.

On the following pages, the lists of opposites can be used as prompters for identifying and discussing feelings.

 ⬥ If you're not certain what to call a particular mood or feeling, describe it as specifically as you can and then give it a made-up name. This will help you to recognize and respond to that feeling more effectively in the future.

 For example, you may go through periods of helplessness during which you feel stupid, lethargic, detached, and almost drugged—a cluster of sensations commonly experienced by prostate cancer patients and their caretakers. To make yourself more aware of this particular cluster of sensations, you might call it the "woollies" (as if you were covered by some sort of thick wool blanket) or the "whelms" (as if you were overwhelmed into passivity).

 ⬥ In addition to describing the feelings that you have during your *waking* life, don't forget to describe the feelings you have during your *dream* life. Very often dreams deal with emotions that we are unable or unwilling to acknowledge while we're awake, even though they may have a major impact on the way we behave. And scientific research has indicated

How DO I Feel

Negative	Positive
denying/disbelieving	accepting/believing
angry	having good will
hateful/hostile	loving/open
fearful	confident
desperate/hopeless	having faith/hopeful
sad/depressed	joyful/elated
incompetent/unable to control	masterful/effective
anxious/panicked	calm/peaceful
exhausted	energized
suicidal	life affirming
grieving/mournful	celebratory
guilty	innocent
shameful	proud
resentful/indignant	grateful/appreciative
engulfed/trapped	free/relieved
disappointed	satisfied
ignored/rejected	acknowledged/approved
indifferent/bored	caring/interested
annoyed	pleased
embarrassed	bold
cowardly	brave
tense/nervous	relaxed
alienated/lonely/isolated	related/united/assisted
disgusted	delighted
confused	enlightened
humiliated	honored
cheated	treated fairly

that people are more likely to have vivid dreams—and troubled sleep—during times of emotional stress than they are at other times.

◊ For recurring feelings, try creating a rating system, using an intensity scale of 1 to 5, with 1 representing the least intensity. For example, if you find yourself repeatedly writing about feeling depressed, you might start rating each day's depression, thus distinguishing between, say, a "level 2" depression one day, and a "level 4" depression another day. This strategy will help you gain control over your feelings, so that you don't overreact to them or inadvertently allow them to escalate.

◊ If you have a great deal of trouble identifying and describing emotions, try creating a "checklist" that you can use each day, at least until you feel more adept. Follow these four steps:

1. Use a lined 8 1/2" x 11" sheet of paper. Along the margin, from the first line to a line halfway down the page, list painful emotions: one per line. Include the ones mentioned above (in the sections dealing with a patient's and a caregiver's emotional reactions), and add: "hurt," "disappointment," "rejection," and "abandonment." Leave space on the line next to each emotion for future comments.

2. The rest of the way down the margin (from halfway down the sheet to the last line on the sheet) list pleasurable emotions or states of being: one per line. Include "joy," "love," "affection," "appreciation," "closeness," "well-being," "hope," "competence," "achievement," "pride," "support," and "gratitude." Leave space next to each emotion or state of being for comments.

3. Make numerous photocopies of this sheet, and put them into a loose-leaf folder.

4. Each day, using one of the sheets, check the emotions that you've felt and briefly describe the circumstances. You

may want to rate how much you felt each emotion on a scale of 1 to 5, one being the least intense.

Breathing for Relaxation

In times of emotional stress, our bodies grow tense and our breathing gets rapid and shallow. As a result, we become increasingly uncomfortable and therefore even more emotionally upset. The following "progressive relaxation" exercise helps to break this escalating spiral of emotional and physical stress. (NOTE: Before trying this exercise, read all of the instructions several times, until you feel that you can remember the exercise adequately without having to consult the text):

1. Lie down in a comfortable place. Breathe easily and regularly. Focus on your breathing. As you inhale, feel your breath bringing peace and calm to every part of your body. As you exhale, feel your breath taking away tensions and troubles. Do this for a few moments.

2. At your next inhalation, point your toes and stretch the bottoms of your feet. Hold your breath and, as you do, hold your feet in the outstretched position. Then gently exhale, and relax your feet. Breathe comfortably for a few moments.

3. At your next inhalation, tighten your leg muscles, and stretch your legs to their fullest downward extension, as if you were trying to pull them out of their hip sockets. Hold this position as you hold your breath, then gently exhale, and relax your legs. Breathe comfortably for a few moments. Feel your legs becoming warm, heavy, and relaxed.

4. When you next inhale, tighten the muscles of your buttocks. Hold this tightness as you hold your breath. Gently exhale, and relax your buttocks. Breathe comfortably for a few moments.

5. When you next inhale, tighten your stomach muscles. Hold this tightness as you hold your breath. Gently

exhale, and relax. Feel the whole lower half of your body becoming heavy, warm, and relaxed.

6. At your next inhalation, make your hands into two fists, and pull your arms straight down, as if you were pulling them out of their sockets. Hold your breath, and hold your hands and arms in this tight position. Then, gently exhale, and relax your arms and hands. Breathe comfortably for a few moments.

7. When you next inhale, pull your head down and touch your chest with your chin. Hold this position as you hold your breath for as long as you can. Then exhale, relaxing your head and your chest muscles. Now, feel your whole body becoming warm, heavy, and relaxed. Breathe comfortably for a few moments.

8. When you next inhale, raise your shoulders up toward your ears, and hold them there as you hold your breath for as long as you can. Then exhale, and relax your head and neck. Breathe comfortably for a few minutes.

9. At your next inhalation, scrunch up your face, tightening all of your facial muscles. Become aware of how much tension you are carrying in your face. Hold this position as you hold your breath for as long as you can. Then exhale, relaxing your muscles and feeling all the tightness dissolve.

10. Breathe comfortably for a while. If there is any part of your body that still feels tense, visualize your breath as a ray of soft warmth that can be directed to that tight place to relax and heal it. Stay in this position for as long as you wish.

11. Think of a code word for the way you feel now, when you are completely relaxed—any pleasant word or sound that comes to mind, regardless of any exact meaning it may have. Practice saying this word to yourself as you feel your whole body being relaxed, warm, and heavy.

Later, recalling this code word can help you summon up these comforting sensations.

You may want to tape-record the above instructions so that you have a tape to play that can guide you step by step through the breathing relaxation. While you're recording, be careful to speak calmly and slowly, allowing several seconds to pass after each sentence and an even longer period after each numbered instruction.

An alternative is to purchase ready-made relaxation tapes from catalogues or stores or order them from us. Some of these tapes follow a similar breath-related procedure to induce relaxation; others offer a "guided visualization," in which the narrator prompts the listener to imagine—and, to some degree, experience—mentally and emotionally soothing scenarios.

6

Choosing among
Treatment Options

⬥ Guidelines for making treatment decisions

⬥ Descriptions and comparisons of the major treatments for prostate cancer

From April 1991, when he was diagnosed, to his death at age fifty-nine on November 21, 1993, the popular television actor Bill Bixby amazed his family, friends, and fans with the sheer intensity of his battle against prostate cancer. It was a multiround prizefight for life that took him through surgery, chemotherapy, experimental hormone treatment, and agonizing personal dilemmas: whether to continue as director of the NBC sitcom *Blossom* (he did) and whether to pursue his romantic interest in the artist Judith Kliban (he did, and they married six weeks before his death). When he was asked by reporters what his most difficult challenge had been throughout the entire ordeal, he replied:

Without question, it was trying to decide what to do about treating the cancer. It's a maddening, mysterious disease. Each case is unique, and you get a bewildering amount of conflicting information and opinions. You have to go through so much of it just by your own instincts.

The bewilderment Bixby experienced is familiar to any patient or caretaker who enters wholeheartedly into decision-making research on prostate cancer treatment. Unfortunately, many patients and caregivers respond to a diagnosis with such panic that they never enter the decision-making process at all.

People vary greatly in their ability—and willingness—to deal with such a matter. A patient's partner may be interested in taking an active, decision-making role, but the patient himself may be more inclined to say, "Whatever you think best, Doc." Some patients say this right away; others wait only until they've had their first shock of bewilderment. They explain it to themselves, their family, and their friends, by saying, "Isn't it a doctor's job to make that decision?" or "*I'm* certainly not qualified to make that decision." Caregivers who don't want to become involved in the decision-making process might declare to their partners, "It's your body, your life, and your decision," or "I'm not going to be the one who says, 'Do this, do that'"; and they might justify their withdrawal by claiming, "I don't want to add any pressure at a time like this," "I don't want that responsibility," or simply "I'm in no state right now to make a rational decision."

Although each person's approach to decision making needs to be respected as his or her personal right, this chapter is designed to encourage you to take as active a role as you can, and to support you in that endeavor. The job of making any treatment decision related to prostate cancer properly belongs to the patient *and* his caregiver, functioning as a team. And so we come to our three main personal recommendations about performing that task:

1. *You and your partner need to work together to make the best possible treatment decision.*

Because you are both intimately involved with the illness, you are both the most qualified people to participate in the decision-making process. If you rush to agree with the diagnosing doctor's recommendation, and the treatment has consequences that you didn't expect or prepare for, it does no good—and it's not fair—to blame the doctor. And you will certainly blame yourselves, as couple after couple interviewed for this book confessed.

Remember, the decision that is made will affect both the patient and you, the primary caregiver, in many ways. It involves not just physical survival but the quality of the lives that are left for each of you to live. The patient, naturally, should have the final word, but as the caregiver, you should—and must—say all that you have to say on the matter that might be helpful. This is not a time for timidity or passing the buck. It's a time when your courage and your contribution can mean more than at any other time in your relationship.

> 2. *In order to make the best possible decision, you need to take it upon yourself to conduct as much research into the decision-making issues as you reasonably can.*

There is almost always time to research the full range of treatment options to some degree before a decision has to be made, and it is always time well spent. No activity related to the illness is more important for you to perform. It's instructive, empowering, and, quite possibly, life saving.

Conducting personal research is not solely a matter of putting yourselves in the best position to choose the most appropriate treatment. It's also a matter of equipping yourselves to go through any treatment and its aftermath as competently and with as much preparation as you can. You must be able to understand what doctors tell you about the patient's case. You must be knowledgeable about the world of treatment in general, so that you can better oversee, evaluate, influence, and improve the professional care the patient receives.

It is our opinion that patients and caregivers of any serious illness, especially an illness like prostate cancer that has so many unknowns, cannot afford to remain passive and uninformed, accepting whatever their doctors say. Some couples get away with their ignorance, but many do not. In a situation with such a high degree of risk attached, why leave even more to chance?

3. Take care to establish goals relating not only to survival but also to quality of life and quantity of resources.

Among the results you want from treatment, sheer survival will, of course, be your top priority. However, you also need to consider the *quality* of the life that survives.

If you look at the label on a bottle of aspirin—or any other over-the-counter medication—you can see a long list of warnings about possible side effects, some minor and some quite serious. It is important to know that every drug and medical or surgical treatment carries with it a "risk factor" and a "likelihood factor." The risk factor refers simply to the individual things that can go wrong (depending, for example, on the side effects of the drug/treatment itself, or on the patient's physical condition, age, or lifestyle). The likelihood factor, attached to each of these risk factors, refers to the probability that it will actually occur.

In considering quality-of-life issues relating to prostate cancer treatments, you, your partner, and your doctor, working together, need to identify the risk factors of various treatments, the likelihood factors attached to these risks in your partner's case, *and* how much you're willing to risk certain likelihoods. The more specific you and your partner are about what *type* of life you want to lead after treatment, the better you can aim for it in your treatment choices and the more assured you can be about getting it. And so you must do some deep soul-searching as well as some serious legwork, so that you can honestly answer very difficult questions like the ones below (some of which apply only to the most advanced stages of prostate cancer or its treatment):

◊ Can the patient go through a potentially long, arduous, and (in some cases) painful recovery period, with the possible need for future treatments? Even if the patient can do so, does he want to?

◊ How big a problem—physically and emotionally— might posttreatment sexual dysfunction really be for each of you? How about loss of sexual desire on the patient's part? How might such a dysfunction or loss impinge on your lifestyle together, or your self-image as individuals?

Through conversations and research, establish as precisely as you can how the patient and you, the primary caretaker, would feel about the nitty-gritty realities of specific problems relating to sex or reproduction:

- ◊ inability to get or maintain a firm erection,

- ◊ the possibilities of using prosthetics to facilitate intercourse,

- ◊ the possibility of relying solely on "nonpenetration" sexual activities,

- ◊ your partner's possible lack of libido, and

- ◊ infertility.

◊ Are you open to joint consultation with a psychologist and/or sex therapist on these matters?

◊ How big a problem—physically and emotionally—might urinary and/or bowel incontinence really be? How about frequent leakage, potentially requiring the constant use of pads? Leakage during sex?

◊ How big a problem—physically and emotionally—might intestinal dysfunction and/or discomfort really be?

◊ What other impacts might each possible treatment's aftermath have on the physical, psychological, and social well-being of the patient? How willing and able are the patient and you to accept these impacts?

◊ What impact might the financial costs associated with each treatment and its aftermath have on your life as a couple?

This last question is an especially tricky issue. It's impossible to put a price on human life, and in many cases, insurance steps in to pay most—if not all—of the treatment expenses themselves. Nevertheless, you need to anticipate the full range of *possible financial* consequences, just to be sure you're not caught off guard.

The average cost of a prostatectomy, for example, can be about $20,000, according to Kit Simpson, a health-policy specialist at the University of North Carolina at Chapel Hill. Treating surgery-related incontinence or impotency could mean another $10,000. Avoiding surgery and waiting until later to treat a more advanced stage of that cancer with a combination of therapies might cost up to $70,000.

And added to all these treatment-related expenses are other, hidden costs: missed days at work, transport to clinics and hospitals, special equipment and furniture. Some couples have had to liquidate their investments or sell their homes—either to pay treatment-related expenses themselves, or to prepare the caregiver for a possible life in the near future as a widow. Such developments can have a significant, negative impact on the couple's quality of life.

Making Quality-of-Life Decisions by Dr. Barbara

A helpful way to arrive at a decision in accord with your inner feelings is to use the following decision-making process developed by Dr. Robert Carkhuff of Carkhuff Associates in Massachusetts. It actually *assists you to* measure the degree to which various solution options meet your needs.

1. Determine what your *values* are—those issues that are really important to you personally. For example, if I were ready to retire and needed to decide whether to live in New York City, Montreal, or Vermont, the values I would list might include: *convenience*, proximity to *friends*. proximity to *family, safety*, proximity to *academic centers, cultural activities*, and *aesthetics*. (By comparison, a values list relating to a prostate cancer treatment decision might, depending on the individual and the case. include: extended survival rate, continence, ability to get an erection, and mobility.)

2. Assign a numerical *weight* to each of these values based on the total number of values listed: the most important

value getting the highest number; and the least important, the lowest number. For example, since I have 7 values listed, I would assign a weight of 7 to the most important, *safety.* and a 1 to the least important, proximity to *family.*

3. To clarify how your values are served by the individual options, assign to each value a *positive or negative measure* for each option, according to the following code (number in parentheses refers to a multiplication factor—see step 5):

$$++ \; = \; \text{very positively (x 2)}$$
$$+ \; \; = \; \text{positively (x 1)}$$
$$0 \; \; = \; \text{negatively (x 0)}$$
$$-- \; = \; \text{very negatively (x -2)}$$

4. Put all this information into a *grid,* as follows (using my example):

Value	Weight (Options)	NY	Mon.	VT
Safety	7	- -	+	++
Aesthetics	6	0	+	++
Convenience	5	+	0	0
Academic Center	4	++	+	0
Friends	3	+	++	+
Cultural Activities	2	++	++	+
Family	1	+	+	+

5. To calculate the *true value* of each option, multiply the weight of each value times the positive or negative measure under each option (see the multiplication factors listed in parentheses in step 3). For example, these are the true values (figures under each option) based on the grid above (step 4):

Value	Weight (Options:	NY	Mon.	VT
Safety	7	−14	+7	+14
Aesthetics	6	0	+6	+12
Convenience	5	+5	0	0

Academic Center	4	+8	+4	0
Friends	3	+3	+6	+3
Cultural Activities	2	+4	+4	+2
Family	1	+1	+1	+1

6. To arrive at your final *ranking*, total each option column. The option with the highest number reflects your "preferred" choice. For example, the true values given above (step 5) yield the following rankings: [I] VT (+32), [2] Montreal (+28), and [3] New York (+7).

In a situation as critical as making a treatment decision for prostate cancer, it's important to get as much information as possible from your research and to be as clear with yourself as you can about your feelings, your priorities, and your options. The type of decision-making process described above should be done only after your research and soul-searching are close to complete.

This initial clarification of your decision-making criteria—including objectives relating to quality of life and quantity of resources—is very challenging, but very necessary. You need to establish some parameters for "trade-offs." For example, is it worth choosing surgery as your best chance to get rid of all of the cancer, if it means that the patient might risk being permanently impotent and incontinent? Is it worth having a treatment that stands a good chance of guaranteeing the patient at least two more years of life, if certain factors are likely to make that life intolerable to the patient?

In the words of one of the health-care authorities interviewed for this book, every decision relating to prostate cancer treatment is a cost-benefit analysis. Unfortunately, you must reconcile yourself right from the start to the fact that there is rarely, if ever, one clear, definitive solution to the situation, but instead numerous options for potential solution.

Seek input from a wide variety of sources.

Even if your diagnosing doctor is an internationally acknowledged expert in his or her field, that doesn't mean that he or she has all the right answers. Certainly an expert's opinion should carry a lot of weight; but keep in mind that prostate cancer is an unusually complicated and mysterious illness. No one person is qualified to speak with equal expertise about all the possible treatment options and ramifications. Every expert is, by necessity, a specialist; and when it comes to prostate cancer, no specialist can offer certainties.

Murray Corwin, a sixty-six-year-old prostate cancer survivor, summarized the situation in a recent interview for UCLA's *Advances* magazine:

> As a [prostate cancer] patient, you're saying, "Gosh, Doctor, if my arteries were clogged, you would recommend a bypass. If my leg were broken, there'd be no question how you try to mend it. What about my prostate cancer?" And the doctor says, "Let's talk about the options."

The best that doctors can do in a case of prostate cancer is to present the patient with treatment choices; and different, equally qualified doctors might well disagree about the possible ways to treat the exact same case. Add to this factor the unique psychology and lifestyle preferences of the individual patient, and the result is a very complex appraisal process before a final treatment decision can be made. This is why effective, ongoing communication among the members of the health-care team—which includes you and your partner, your doctor and other professionals is essential.

Be sure to speak to a number of specialists in different areas pertaining to the patient's illness: surgeons, radiologists, authorities in hormone treatment for prostate cancer, and chemotherapists who are knowledgeable about prostate cancer (not all chemotherapists are). And don't ignore the mental and emotional specialists, such as psychiatrists, psychologists, sex therapists. They cannot only provide you with specific guidance, they can also make you more confident in general about your decision-making capabilities.

Don't be discouraged if all this activity seems daunting on paper. Remember simply to do the best you can each day, and to respect your personal limits as you go along. As laborious and perplexing as it may be to conduct this kind of decision-making process, most patients and caretakers *can* do it, and do it effectively, with the help of others.

In 1991, Dr. Barrie R. Cassileth, formerly associate professor at the University of Pennsylvania School of Medicine and now president of her own consulting firm, conducted a study of patient decision-making among 159 men, averaging age seventy, with previously untreated Stage D prostate cancer. Speaking to urologists about the results of this study, Cassileth had this to say about encouraging patients to take a more active role in making treatment decisions:

> Patients can be educated and informed about their treatment options, and with the guidance of their physicians and families, they are able to make decisions with which they remain satisfied over time. Full patient participation is an achievable, practical goal.
>
> Medicine is changing so dramatically. It is crucial to keep patients informed. They are eager to know about the disease and to play an active role in their treatment. And it is their right.

Finally, make a concerted effort to talk with other patients and caretakers about their experiences. These contacts can give you invaluable insights into "quality-of-life" issues. To find people with whom you can talk, ask among your family members and friends and investigate local support groups (see the "Resources" section in chapter 10). Preferably, consult with patients who are—or were—in a similar situation: relatively the same diagnosis, age, overall physical condition, economic bracket, lifestyle, and geographic locale.

Get as much help as you can in your research effort.

Divide the research effort into separate tasks: e.g., locating and reading certain books, locating and recruiting certain people with whom to consult, establishing the cost-range of certain services or treatments. Then, assign trusted, competent family members and friends to do some of the research for you or with you. Also, enlist the special attention of a friendly librarian or any other professional who is better equipped than you are to perform potentially helpful research functions.

When researching books and other literature, keep in mind that what you're reading may reflect a biased point of view. For example, a urologist or clinical investigator is more likely to publish his or her "good" results than the failures, and the studies he or she quotes to support a thesis may not actually be as impressive as they seem. When in doubt, it's a good idea to ask your doctor or another qualified authority what he or she thinks about the credibility of the material.

Don't give up, and pursue all leads.

Although the time you and your partner have to make a decision about prostate cancer treatment may be somewhat limited, the illness typically develops very slowly, so it s almost always possible to take at least *some* time to research and weigh your options. You will feel better about the illness experience as a whole if you allow yourself to do whatever you can in the time available. Yes, you will probably experience fatigue, bewilderment, and outright panic at certain moments, but your perseverance can make a great deal of positive difference. Consider these two experiences volunteered by people interviewed for this book:

(Wife of a patient in his seventies, after the doctor suggested a hormone treatment that would extend the patient's life an estimated eighteen months):

> My husband is a very positive man, but he was so flabbergasted by the prognosis, he didn't ask [the doctor] any questions. It's that father-son relationship the [older] patient often has with the [younger] doctor that gets in the way. They chat, but they don't touch the scary parts.
>
> Then, at a meeting of Us Too [a prostate cancer support group], people talked about new drugs we didn't know about. My husband went to his doctor and

mentioned these new drugs, and the doctor was cordial
and put him on them. If we hadn't mentioned them to
the doctor, he probably wouldn't have prescribed them.
Being put on the new drugs changed the whole prognosis. It was no longer eighteen months that my husband
had open to him—but indefinitely longer.

(Patient age sixty-seven, after the doctor suggested a radical prostatectomy):

I had just about made up my mind to choose surgery
when my wife read some articles on European medical
practices that mentioned cryosurgery. I learned all I
could about it—including that it was less dangerous,
required a shorter hospital stay, and had fewer side
effects—and found out the hospitals in the U.S. where
it's done. One of the doctors I'd interviewed before I
knew about cryosurgery called to find out what I'd
decided, and when I told him about cryosurgery, he
said, "That's a smart decision. I went to study about
cryosurgery recently." So why hadn't he mentioned it
before? I assume because it's still classified as experimental, although insurance companies are paying for it.

The point made by these two stories is *not* that doctors are
remiss in their duties. Doctors can only advise what they believe,
based on their professional expertise, is the best course of action.
Nor is the point that patients should take matters into their own
hands, especially based on something that another, nonprofes-
sional person tells them. What turns out to work in one case (e.g.,
cryosurgery, which is, in fact, a controversial therapy still considered investigational), may not work at all in another case; and
patients shouldn't feel as if they have to "clutch at straws."

The point of these two stories is that patients and their caregivers are well advised to become involved in the decision-
making process themselves, and to pursue any promising leads.
After all, they are the ones who have the broadest perspective on
the life at stake, and the ultimate responsibility for making the
decision. This doesn't mean that they should make any final

judgments without first discussing every issue thoroughly with their doctor and securing his or her cooperation. That's an integral part of "pursuing any promising leads." But it does mean that they should keep an eye and an ear out for any new questions to ask their doctor.

Keep in touch with your feelings.

Throughout the decision-making process, pay close attention to how you react *emotionally* to certain options, as well as how you react intellectually. One of your best guides in making any final treatment decision can be what Bill Bixby called "your instincts" (in the statement quoted at the beginning of this chapter). This isn't merely what is popularly known as a "gut reaction." Rather, it is a deep personal feeling that remains consistent over time, or that builds over time, telling you that one option is more suitable for you than another.

Following are brief overviews of each of the major treatment options. These overviews provide you with all the data that you need for an initial orientation. However, given the rapid rate at which prostate cancer treatment is changing and the lag time between the writing and reading of this book, it will be necessary to gather the most up-to-date information before reaching your final decision. Instead, these overviews are designed solely to help you begin your research.

In considering any information given about specific treatments, you need to be especially careful not to attach too much credibility or significance to statistics. In general, statistics relating to serious illness are psychologically comforting because they appear to provide a concrete, quantifiable basis for making personal decisions. However, survival and side-effect rates for prostate cancer are, at best, only approximate measures of what seems to be occurring within a very broad category of people. Every individual is different, and a given statistic may have nothing to do with that individual. The statistical ranges offered below for each of the major treatment options incorporate statistics published by the most-often-quoted sources in the field, including the American Cancer Society and Medicare records.

Stage-by-Stage Treatment Options

Stage of Cancer	Common Treatment Options (no order of preference)
Stages A/T1 and B/T2 (confined to prostate)	watchful waiting; surgery or radiation
Stage C/T3 or T4 (spread to surrounding areas)	radiation and/or hormone therapy
Stage D/N+ or M+ (widespread in body)	radiation and/or hormone therapy and/or chemotherapy

Watchful Waiting

Let's begin by considering the most conservative approach to dealing with prostate cancer, which is, in essence, to do nothing, at least for a while. Within the medical community and the popular press, the phrase *watchful waiting* refers to the policy of initially withholding treatment in an effort to avoid, if at all possible, potential trauma, complications, and adverse aftereffects—especially in regard to the two most commonly prescribed treatments: surgery to remove the prostate (radical prostatectomy) or radiation to arrest or destroy the cancer (both of these therapies are discussed individually below). Instead, the cancer is monitored through periodic testing to determine: (a) if, over time, its rate of growth or quality of change more evidently warrants treatment; and, if so, (b) what specific type of treatment is apparently the most advisable.

As discussed in chapter 1, watchful waiting is becoming an increasingly popular strategy. It appeals to patients of all ages with early-stage, localized cancer that is well differentiated; but it's particularly attractive to men over seventy, for whom any sort of treatment poses more discomfort with less chance of prolonging life.

However, since watchful waiting represents an ever stronger challenge to the standard modes of treatment, it has also become an increasingly controversial strategy. At present, a high percentage of U.S. doctors are willing to concede that watchful waiting may be a viable option for most men over seventy with early-stage cancers, but they draw the line at recommending it for younger men.

Among all the choices to be made after a diagnosis, the decision to go—or not to go—for watchful waiting can be the most difficult. To begin to get a reasonably balanced picture of the issues at stake, we need to look more carefully at both sides of the controversy. In your own situation of dealing with early-stage prostate cancer and wondering about watchful waiting, you need to keep in mind that there is no definitive treatment for the illness and that there are many quality-of-life considerations. This means that your *informed* choice—after much discussion with a number of qualified proponents of each side of the issue—is as legitimate and defensible as any single doctor's recommendation.

Arguments For Watchful Waiting

To date, the strongest arguments for watchful waiting are made in a study published in *The Journal of the American Medical Association*. In this study, medical scientists with the Prostate Patient Outcomes Research Team reviewed all the scientific literature on the subject and generated statistical models of how patients of all ages are likely to fare in two different scenarios: if they choose to treat an early-stage cancer with surgery or radiation, or if they choose simply to watch and wait. In most cases, the team could find no clear benefit in choosing the former scenario over the latter. Their conclusion was as follows: Since prostate cancer is usually slow growing and may stay localized for years and even decades, most patients with an early-stage diagnosis will probably die of other causes before their cancer can grow to life-threatening proportions.

Dr. Craig Fleming of Oregon Health Science University in Portland, a team member, commented to *New York Times* reporter Natalie Angier:

> The most important part of our study is to let patients know they truly do have an alternative to surgery or radiation therapy. . . . In terms of preserving longevity

and achieving the best quality of life, in many cases watchful waiting may equal the outcomes obtained from either of the more invasive treatments.

According to the report, the situation for patients over seventy years old with prostate cancer especially favors watchful waiting. At that time of life, the risks involved in surgery or radiation outweigh the potential benefit of a longer life span—an increase that the report estimates at less than six months on the average. In the case of patients under age seventy, only those with very large and aggressive tumors, the kind that are most inclined to spread quickly beyond the prostate itself, are considered likely to benefit from surgery or radiation. And even among these cases, quality-of-life issues may tip the patient's decision in favor of watchful waiting. The report concludes that the average increase in life span gained by such patients who opt for surgery or radiation is less than four years, and the risk of posttreatment impotence or incontinence is relatively high.

The report also points out that watchful waiting is far more commonly advised by European doctors than by their American counterparts, and yet there are no measurable differences in longevity among patients with similar types of prostate cancer on either side of the Atlantic. The report ends on a highly confrontational note:

> We expect that many clinicians will find the results of this decision analysis discordant with the view that radical prostatectomy and radiation therapy offer a definite improvement in outcomes for men with localized prostate cancer. Based on conversations with clinicians, our review of the medical literature, the findings of our Medicare claims analysis, and calls for the increasing use of screening for early detection of prostate cancer, it is evident that the prevailing patterns of care in the United States favor invasive treatment of prostate cancer. However, in over two decades during which these treatments have been used, only one randomized clinical trial, of limited power, has been performed to assess the efficacy of these treatments

compared with watchful waiting. If the medical community were to apply the same standards of safety and efficacy required for approval of new drugs to the use of invasive treatments for prostate cancer, it is likely that neither radical prostatectomy nor radiation therapy would be approved for this indication....

Arguments Against Watchful Waiting

As mentioned before, most doctors would agree that watchful waiting is an option well worth considering for a patient over seventy with early-stage cancer, although in certain cases surgery or radiation might still be their principal recommendation. The controversy lies in how appropriate watchful waiting is for a patient under age seventy with early-stage cancer.

Dr. Willet F. Whitmore of Memorial Sloan-Kettering Cancer Center in New York City sums up the prevailing argument against watchful waiting for patients in this younger age group:

Even though we're uncertain about the efficacy of invasive treatment, I would advise some sort of treatment in younger men. If somebody is going to live another fifteen or twenty years, he may well run into problems if he decides against treatment.

Dr. Abraham T. K. Crockett, president of the American Urological Association, concurs:

When prostate cancer is diagnosed while it is still confined to the prostate gland, the cure rate with surgery is high. But once the malignancy has spread, successful treatment becomes extremely difficult. Therefore, watchful waiting may not be a prudent course of action for many middle-aged men diagnosed with prostate cancer.

In response to the observation that European doctors recommend watchful waiting far more often than American doctors, many medical experts point out that a far greater percentage of European health-care expenses are regulated and subsidized by the government, therefore predisposing European physicians to recommend the more financially conservative policy of watchful waiting when they can do so. These same experts add that we can't be certain precisely why prostate cancer patients on either side of the Atlantic have the same survival rate, despite the difference in preferred treatment recommendations. Therefore, it is not necessarily an indication that watchful waiting, on the whole, is as beneficial for treating prostate cancer as surgery or radiation.

Regarding the issue of whether it is justifiable to recommend invasive treatments without first subjecting these treatments to proper clinical trials, most authorities insist that putting a moratorium on such treatments until they can be tested against watchful waiting controls would be grossly inhumane. Although there are no doubt a number of patients who undergo surgery or radiation when they might have done just as well or better with watchful waiting, these authorities argue that a much bigger problem is the number of men who do *not* get surgery or radiation when they need it and, as a result, risk death.

Meanwhile, a major clinical trial involving thousands of patients—some given surgery after diagnosis and an equal number left to watchful waiting—has just begun in Sweden and Finland, and the U.S. Department of Veteran Affairs is considering undertaking its own similar trial. Results from these studies, however, will not be available for at least a decade, after a sufficient amount of time has passed to measure long-range outcomes.

According to Dr. Michael Droller, watchful waiting is probably most appropriate for a patient with a total *Gleason score* of 2–4, a negative digital rectal examination, and an age of seventy or over, or who has a medical condition that allows prediction of a less than ten-year life expectancy. Many patients above the age of seventy will elect to have the least invasive treatment and often will choose radiation. Patients below that age of seventy who have a *Gleason score* >2–4 should be encouraged to consider some form of treatment, since a majority of them will experience progressive disease over the course of ten years, at which point it may be more difficult to control or cure their disease.

Also, the means by which watchful waiting is accomplished needs to be clarified. PSA levels and digital rectal examination at three to six-month intervals are important. However, it's equally important to consider repeat biopsy if the PSA has risen. Patients should be made aware that they are at risk for progressive disease in the setting of watchful waiting.

Radical Prostatectomy

Description: The prostate gland is completely removed by surgery of one type or another with the goal of curing the disease. The surgery may be performed by two different approaches: retropubic (through the lower abdomen) or perineal (through the space between the scrotum and the anus).

Another surgical procedure that does not remove the entire prostate (i.e., is not a radical prostatectomy) and is not curative is transurethral resection or TURP. Cancerous tissue is removed from the prostate, using an instrument that is inserted through the urethra. This relieves symptoms (such as painful or problematic urination) in advance of further treatment or in cases when age or illness prohibits a radical prostatectomy. Some degree of stress urinary incontinence should be expected, but it should not be sufficiently severe to seriously affect a patient's quality of life. Many physicians have suggested that radical prostatectomy is probably the best choice for patients with clinically organ-confined prostate cancer who are below the age of sixty-five.

Common Usage: Stage A/T1, B2, or early C/T3 or T4 cancers; especially for men who are relatively young (forty to sixty).

Side Effects: possible incontinence (less likely if the surgery is retropubic), impotency, surgical damage to healthy tissue in surrounding area.

Surgery is the treatment of choice for early-stage localized cancers. Doctors like it because it provides the surest chance of a complete cure, and patients like it because it's relatively quick and convenient, not to mention the fact that it satisfies the latent wish to simply "get rid of the whole thing."

Nevertheless, surgery to remove the prostate gland is a major operation with potentially far-reaching, irreversible consequences. Just how involved it gets depends upon the particular type of surgery, the overall health of the patient, the skill of the surgical team, and luck. In general, the operation itself may last anywhere from two to four hours, may demand a considerable amount of transfused blood (preferably autodonated—i.e., taken from the patient—ahead of time), and may require a fairly lengthy recovery period: typically five days in the hospital, but perhaps up to two weeks if there are complications, followed by up to three weeks of home-based convalescence. During the home-based convalescence, the patient can usually move around freely as long as he avoids strenuous activity that involves lifting or twisting. He may even be able to return to his job, if it's sedentary. The catheter inserted at the time of surgery is usually removed two to three weeks after surgery.

Many factors go into determining which type of surgery is more appropriate for an individual patient: retropubic or perineal surgery. Overall, retropubic surgery has some advantages over perineal in reducing the risk of impotence or incontinence. Perineal surgery, however, is less physically taxing. The removal of the gland itself is easier. The resulting incision is less uncomfortable (in retropubic surgery, the incision extends from the navel to the pubic bone, making it much longer and therefore slightly more subject to irritation). Also, the convalescent period is substantially shorter. Thus, perineal surgery is often preferred for older patients.

Retropubic surgery is often chosen because it permits the removal and examination of the pelvic lymph nodes, to which prostate cancer often spreads. In certain cases, the nodes may already have been removed by laparoscopic or open pelvic dissection, so this advantage is not a factor. Sometimes, retropubic surgery is performed just to check the lymph nodes, followed by perineal surgery to remove the prostate gland. In these situations, surgeons usually choose to perform the prostatectomy only if the lymph nodes are clear of cancer, thus indicating that the cancer has not spread beyond the prostate; otherwise, a different form of therapy is pursued.

The most significant advance in radical prostatectomy in recent years has been the development of so-called "nerve-sparing" retropubic surgery, which greatly reduces the risk of postoperative impotence. Whether it can be performed on a specific patient depends on the nature and spread of his cancer.

Nerve-sparing surgery was pioneered by Dr. Patrick Walsh, director of the James Buchanan Brady Urological Institute at Johns Hopkins Medical School in Baltimore, Maryland. The story is worth recounting for the insights it gives into the complex nature of prostate surgery.

During the late 1970s, Walsh was performing radical prostatectomies in the traditional manner, and he was greatly disturbed about the then almost certain side effects of incontinence and impotence. If a few men managed to escape these side effects, he reasoned, then there must be a way that more men could. One major trouble with the operation was that it featured a great deal of bleeding. Suction tubes simply weren't able to drain away enough blood to provide superior visibility, and so surgeons had to rely to some extent simply on what they felt. "You were working blind," Walsh recalled in a 1993 interview for *Atlantic Monthly* magazine. "If you thought about it, it would scare you out of your wits. The blood prevented you from seeing what on earth you were doing there."

Walsh studied the blood-flow problem and figured out where and how to pinch off veins so that the prostate gland and its environs remained much more visible during the operation. This resulted in a significantly higher percentage of surgical prostate removals that could avoid slicing through the nearby urethral sphincter, the major cause of postoperative incontinence.

But this still left the problem of postoperative impotence. So little was known at the time about the prostate-related mechanics of getting an erection, and for good reason: Anatomical studies are usually performed on cadavers, and the prostate gland is enmeshed in the type of fat-laden tissue that is destroyed in the embalming process.

In 1981, Walsh conferred with Dr. Peter Donker, a retired Dutch urologist, who had discovered that still-born infants make excellent subjects for prostate study, since their prostate-related nerves are much larger and the fat-laden tissue is much thinner. Studying such a cadaver, Walsh found that the nerve bundles obviously responsible for an erection lay *outside* the prostate itself and were connected to it by a thin, scarcely visible blanket of tissue that was no doubt often cut through, inadvertently, during surgery. He theorized that lifting this blanket of tissue away from the route of surgery, if at all possible, would minimize damage to the nerve bundles and help preserve potency; and subsequent trial operations proved him correct.

Today, nerve-sparing retropubic surgery does not guarantee that potency will be preserved. It clearly offers the opportunity for this to happen, and it appears that it actually does happen more often than with other kinds of prostatectomies (although no scientific proof yet exists). Unfortunately, not every patient is a candidate for it. The nerve-sparing operation has been suggested to permit preservation of potency. Although there are substantial claims of a satisfactory outcome using this approach, the claims have never been appropriately validated. Even presumed preservation of the neurovascular bundles has not necessarily been associated with preservation of full erectile function.

Regarding radical prostatectomy surgery as a whole, statistics on mortality rates and the likelihood of incontinence or impotency vary widely from source to source. Overall, the most-often-quoted numbers suggest that only 1 percent of patients under age seventy-five and only 2 percent of patients age seventy-five and older actually die of the operation itself (although 7 to 10 percent of the latter group suffer serious surgery-related complications such as heart failure). In all age groups, the five-year survival rate after surgery is estimated to be the highest for any therapy—around 85 to 95 percent (depending on the source).

Also in all age groups, 80 to 90 percent of patients are incontinent immediately afterward, but up to 90 percent of these patients regain full continence within twelve weeks (50 percent within five weeks). Among the 10 percent who do not regain full continence, 5 to 8 percent rely on pads to handle stress-related incontinence.

The chances of surgery patients under age sixty-five retaining their potency are generally quoted as 35 to 60 percent (the younger the patient and the lower grade the cancer, the more favorable the odds). Speaking only of his own practice, Walsh claims that nerve-sparing surgery preserves potency in 90 percent of his patients under age fifty, 75 percent of his patients under age fifty-nine, and 60 percent of his patients under age sixty-nine.

However, his particular pool of patients may not be representative of the patient population in general.

Other forms of surgery currently under clinical trial (and therefore still considered "experimental" or "investigational") are:

- ◊ *Cryosurgery:* An instrument called a "cryoprobe" is used to infuse the prostate with super-cooled nitrogen, thereby (hopefully) destroying it. The procedure causes no bleeding and often requires just an overnight stay in the hospital. It has not yet been proven to be curative.

- ◊ *Laser surgery:* Laser surgery is already used to treat benign prostate hyperplasia (BPH); and in recent years, some doctors have been experimenting with using laser surgery, guided by ultrasound imaging, to remove the entire prostate in cases of cancer. Other clinical trials have been combining laser surgery with transurethral resection (TURP): first, TURP is employed in an effort to get rid of most of the organ, followed by laser surgery to trim away—with better accuracy—any remaining tissue. To date, this investigational therapy has prompted even more controversy than cryosurgery, mainly on the grounds of measurement accuracy.

- ◊ *Ultrasound surgery:* Transrectal ultrasound first establishes the area of cancerous tissue to be cut, then bombards that area with waves of tissue-destroying intensity. This therapy is in the very early stages of experimentation.

- ◊ *Robot surgery:* A precision-controlled robotic surgical instrument cuts a pattern established by an earlier internal scan of the patient's lower abdomen. Like ultrasound surgery, this therapy is in the very early stages of experimentation.

External Radiation Therapy

Description: High-energy radiation is focused into a beam that is directed onto the pelvic area and hopefully destroys or deactivates the tumor in the prostate.

Common Usage: Stages B/T2 or C/T3 or T4 cancers.

Side Effects: impotence, "collateral" damage to healthy cells and tissue, irritation to the bladder causing frequent and/or painful urination (also, within the treatment period, possible fatigue, nausea, diarrhea, skin eruptions, urination problems, and rectal bleeding). Incontinence isn't as much of a problem with radiation as is urinary irritability and frequency. The development of impotence may be higher than 40 percent, but the effects of age may be important.

Prescribed for patients whose cancer is confined to a fairly small area (preferably, but not necessarily, localized to the prostate gland), external radiation therapy is the first-choice alternative for men who would prefer not to have surgical treatment. Typically, it is applied on an outpatient basis for a period of approximately seven weeks (up to five days a week) by any one of several different types of radiation machines. One thing you will want to clarify before making final therapy decisions is the treatment schedule that you would be expected to follow:

◊ How long will the treatments take, individually and collectively?

◊ Can they be scheduled during the day according to your convenience?

◊ What happens if you miss a treatment?

The external radiation procedure itself is painless, and 60 to 75 percent of patients escape any significant discomfort from side effects. For the rest of the patients, the discomfort can usually be alleviated with medication. Almost always, treatment-related symptoms cease to occur after the therapy has run its full course (typically, a time period of less than three months).

Because the high-energy rays used in this therapy cannot be targeted toward the cancerous tissue with precision, nearby healthy cells are inevitably damaged at the same time; but the healthy cells are much better able to recover. In most cases, the radiation doses are small enough and sufficiently spread out over time that the healthy cells ultimately survive and the cancer cells do not.

In early-stage prostate cancer, radiation therapy can sometimes cure the disease. Indeed, its estimated five-year survival rate for early-stage cancer comes close to the rate for surgery: about 75 to 85 percent (compared with 85 to 95 percent for surgery). Otherwise, one of two things may happen:

1. The external radiation simply arrests the disease and prevents it from spreading, which, if successful, is all that is needed for the patient to maintain normal good health and life expectancy; or

2. Cancer cells that are not destroyed by the radiation cause the cancer to spread, ultimately resulting in the death of the patient (unless further rounds of therapy stop or kill the cancer in time). Assuming the cancer does continue to spread, it may grow at a much slower rate than it would have without treatment, thus making the treatment responsible for prolonging the patient's life. However, this possibility has not actually been proven and in fact would be very difficult to prove. (Some scientists speculate that, in some cases, radiation may even make certain components of the cancer grow faster.)

For midstage cancer, when surgery is often not advised, the five-year (at least) survival rate for external radiation patients drops to about 55 to 65 percent.

Radiation is less likely to cause incontinence or impotence than surgery is. There is still substantial controversy regarding the recurrence rate following radiation therapy in those patients who are younger and are expected to have a greater than ten-year survival. Several changes in this approach include the development of a 3-D conformal radiation, the use of preradiation, and the possible use of postradiation hormonal therapy. How these affect overall freedom of disease and cause-specific survival is not yet known.

Brachytherapy

Description: Also known as "internal (or interstitial) radiation," brachytherapy involves inserting radioactive "seeds" directly into the prostate, where they emit rays that, hopefully, destroy or deactivate the tumor.

Common Usage: Stages B2 or C/T3 or T4 cancer.

Side Effects: possible incontinence, impotence (also, within the treatment period, possible nausea, fatigue, diarrhea, bladder or rectal irritation).

According to Dr. Michael Droller, brachytherapy (radioactive seed implantation) has attracted great interest, and many patients are now opting for this approach. Long-term survival data is not available. Disease-specific survival appears to match that of surgery, stage for stage, although median and mean intervals are not yet available. The means by which the radioactive seeds are implanted is important. Sonographic guidance appears to be of value because the prostate may change its position during respiration, and reliance on template alone may not be sufficient to achieve accurate dosimetry. The potential irregularity of seed placement probably led to the many failures that were experienced when brachytherapy was first introduced over thirty years ago. In many instances brachytherapy is supplemented by preimplant hormonal therapy as well as by postimplant external radiation. The efficacy of this approach remains to be determined.

Brachytherapy is used somewhat more conservatively than external radiation; typically, it is a treatment reserved for early-stage cancer. Minute capsules filled with radioactive material are implanted in the prostate gland by means of a relatively minor surgical operation that cuts through the perineum.

Often the surgery is performed on an outpatient basis; but sometimes a hospital stay of up to two or three days is involved, to ensure that adverse side effects are expediently managed or that an older patient recovers more comfortably from the overall trauma of surgery. The capsules inserted into the prostate remain there permanently and imperceptibly, but they emit their strong, cancer-destroying rays for only about a year at the most.

The idea of harboring a radioactive substance within one's body is still daunting to many people, who immediately associate any mention of "radioactivity" with atomic-bomb fallout, the Three Mile Island meltdown, Chernobyl, and glow-in-the-dark science-fiction mutants. The type of radioactivity associated with brachytherapy does not belong in this catalogue of horrors. In itself, it poses no threat to the patient's health or well-being, nor is it capable of producing any physical sensations (such as heat or knifelike pain from the rays—two common misconceptions).

Possible side effects associated with the brachytherapy treatment itself are similar in kind to those associated with external radiation. However, they are much less likely to happen during brachytherapy; and if they do occur, they are generally milder. Brachytherapy patients very seldom experience side effects beyond three months after implantation.

Estimated survival rates for brachytherapy patients are roughly the same as those for external radiation. Rates of incontinence and impotence are lower in the case of brachytherapy: around 3 percent for incontinence and 10 to 25 percent for impotence. These rates vary somewhat according to the particular radioactive substance contained in the implant. The rates just given are associated with iodine 125, the most commonly used substance. Even lower rates are attributed to the combination of iodine and palladium 103 (sometimes used in conjunction with X-ray treatment).

Hormone Therapy (Medical)

Description: Medicines are administered to prevent the release, or counter the action, of male hormones such as testosterone, which promote the growth of prostate cancer cells.

Common Usage: Stages C/T3 or T4 or D/N+ or M+ cancers. (For early-stage cancers, so-called Combination Hormonal Therapy, or CHT, is sometimes used.)

Side Effects: likely impotence; possible loss of libido, "feminization"—e.g., breast development, malaise, hot flashes, stomach/intestinal discomfort, vomiting, cardiovascular problems.

An estimated 90 percent of prostate cancers are stimulated by male hormones. Thus, for more advanced cancers or for older patients who may not be able to sustain the rigors of surgery or radiation, medical hormone therapy aimed at preventing or counteracting the production of male hormones is the most commonly recommended treatment. An alternative hormone therapy is surgical: the removal of the testicles, which are the primary producers of male hormones (see the next section: "Hormone Therapy [Surgical]").

Hormone therapy can't cure the cancer, but it can slow or stop the cancer's further development. Sometimes it can even reduce the size of an existing growth. In any event, the patient usually feels better as a result of the therapy than he did before, and his life expectancy is usually prolonged.

Medical hormone treatment almost always continues for the rest of the patient's life, so treatment-related side effects are always a possibility. Depending on the specific type of medical hormone therapy used, patients have at least a fifty-fifty chance of never experiencing any side effects. For those who do, medication can often help (except with such side effects as impotence and "feminization"). Feminization may be arrested, and other side effects can almost certainly be lessened or eliminated, if the therapy is reduced in intensity or discontinued; however, this will most likely increase the chances of the cancer spreading.

Medical hormone therapy is a very rapidly changing field, with new advances being made at a faster rate than in any other type of prostate cancer therapy. At present, however, doctors generally advise one of two basic therapeutic strategies: *female hormone therapy* or *LH-RH therapy*. Let's look at each one separately.

> *Female hormone therapy* involves the administration of a female hormone (usually estrogen, but possibly another, such as DES) to reduce the production of testosterone. The patient takes the hormone in the form of daily tablets. Possible adverse side effects associated specifically with estrogen therapy include cardiovascular problems, water retention (bloating), stomach upset, and nausea.

LH-RH therapy is a more recently developed form of medical hormone therapy that features a drug technically known as a luteinizing hormone-releasing hormone or LH-RH analogue. The ultimate effect of the drug is to lower testosterone production in the testicles almost to zero. It is administered in one of two ways, depending on the specific situation: either through a daily injection by the patient (or the patient's caregiver) or through a monthly injection—with a larger-bore needle—by a urologist in his or her office.

Sometimes the LH-RH drug is administered in combination with an *antiandrogen* drug in an attempt to increase the potential effectiveness of LH-RH therapy. Unfortunately, the antiandrogen drug can produce side effects of its own, including feminization, nausea, and diarrhea.

Compared to female hormone therapy, there is much less risk of feminization with LH-RH therapy— even LH-RH therapy combined with an antiandrogen drug. There is also less chance of suffering from the other side effects associated with female hormones (although the patient can still experience impotence, loss of libido, and hot flashes). For these reasons, patients who are candidates for medical hormone therapy are increasingly attracted to LH-RH treatment, although in some cases it is not as reliable as female hormone treatment.

Combination Hormonal Therapy (CHT) refers to a highly controversial treatment strategy for early-stage prostate cancer. During the first six months after diagnosis, hormones are administered to the patient before any other action is taken. Afterward, biopsies are periodically performed in order to determine if the situation warrants further treatment and, if so, what particular treatment is warranted.

The controversy regarding CHT is similar to the "watchful waiting" controversy discussed earlier in this chapter. Indeed, the two are directly related.

Many experts believe that the CHT approach to treating early-stage cancer is too conservative, potentially allowing the cancer to spread when it might have been stopped or even cured by more aggressive treatment right away. Others counterargue that CHT offers the patient a better chance to continue living a "normal" life—free from the possibly negative consequences of more invasive or injurious treatments.

Hormone Therapy (Surgical)

Description: Commonly referred to as "castration," surgical hormone therapy involves the removal of the testicles (bilateral orchiectomy) in order to stop their production of male hormones, which promote the growth and spread of prostate cancer cells.

Common Usage: Stages C/T3 or T4 or D/N+ or M+ cancers.

Side Effects: infertility, possible impotence, "feminization" (e.g., breast development), loss of libido.

The surest way to stop production of testosterone by the testicles is to remove them altogether, and this is often advised for patients with advanced stages of cancer or patients who are too old or too ill to withstand the rigors of other forms of treatment. The treatment is palliative rather than curative. After the testicles are removed, small amounts of testosterone will still be produced by the adrenal gland, but the stimulant effect on the cancer will be significantly reduced. On the whole, surgical hormone therapy is more often, and more dramatically, successful than medical hormone therapy.

The surgery itself is a relatively simple, painless, onetime procedure: an incision is made through the scrotum and the testicles are quickly and easily cut out. In many cases, the surgery can be performed on an outpatient basis with a local anesthetic, but sometimes hospitalization is required.

For many patients and their caregivers, the concept of surgical hormone therapy is immediately repellent, implying that the patient will no longer be a "man." In fact, most patients who choose to have their testicles surgically removed do not experience "feminization" problems (such as breast enlargement) or, indeed, any of the other physical side effects specifically linked to drug-based therapies.

Furthermore, the removal of the testicles in itself does not always lead to impotence. Some men continue to have erections naturally, just as they did before the surgery. Those men who are impotent after the operation (admittedly, the majority) can produce erections with the help of an implantable penile prosthesis, which means that they may still be able to achieve—and produce—sexual satisfaction through penetration. (See chapter 8 for more information on this prosthesis.) For some patients and their caregivers, sexual satisfaction through penetration may not be an important quality-of-life issue, in which case surgical hormone therapy may be a less threatening alternative.

A bigger problem than impotence may be the patient's loss of libido. According to Dr. Stephen N. Rous of the Medical University of South Carolina, author of *The Prostate Book*, most men who have their testicles removed will experience a loss of sexual desire. In these cases, the patient needs to go through a significant mental and emotional readjustment either to recover his erotic feelings for his partner, or to accept that he will never experience these feelings in quite the same way.

Referring to patients who are concerned about loss of libido and therefore have trouble committing to surgical hormone therapy even though they know it's the wisest course of action, Rous comments:

> . . . what seems to be anathema to most men about bilateral orchiectomy is almost unrelated to intercourse itself and strikes at the very core of maleness: emasculation in an intellectual sense. . . . I have found that most patients will ultimately go along with bilateral orchiectomy . . . once they realize that their own self-image and self-worth are not totally contained in their testes.

Nor are their feelings for their partners totally contained in their testes. For suggestions on how to reromanticize relationships, regardless of any physical limitations in sexual functioning and despite loss of libido, see chapter 9.

Chemotherapy

Description: Drugs are administered that have a toxic effect on cancer cells, thereby reducing the extent of the disease and lessening or eliminating the symptoms.

Common Usage: Stage D/N+ or M+ cancers

Side Effects: possible nausea, physical weakness, weight loss, hair loss, diarrhea, increased risk of infection, decreased blood-clotting ability

Chemotherapy is a very strong therapy that is systemic in nature: i.e., the drugs circulate throughout the entire body. Therefore, chemotherapy is capable of producing a wide variety of discomforting side effects. All of these side effects—including hair loss—are reversible if the therapy is reduced in intensity or discontinued.

Because of its potentially powerful toxic effect on the body, chemotherapy is a "last resort" strategy usually reserved for the most-advanced-stage cancer. The specific type of drug—or drug combination—used varies widely from patient to patient, as does the dosage amount and frequency, which must be controlled very precisely. Depending on the situation, the drug is administered either in pill form or through injection into a vein or muscle.

For many patients, chemotherapy simply does not hold much promise. For others, it may offer limited, but welcome, relief from the symptoms of advanced prostate cancer. It rarely stops the spread of cancer altogether and never results in a cure.

Other Therapies

When positive margins occur after radical prostaectomy, or if the PSA does not decrease to undetectable levels, some have suggested that adjunctive external radiation may facilitate control of disease or possibly convert what may have been an inadequate treatment to a cure. As yet this has not been validated. However the concept of applying external radiation (which has not resulted in any additional morbidity) is attractive on the assumption that remaining cancer cells may be amenable to radiotherapy cure.

Adjunctive hormonal therapy can be reserved if and when there is evidence of recurrent disease at distant sites.

It's important to understand what "undetectable" means in terms of PSA determination. There are may studies that have described "undetectable" as anything less than 0.5 ng/ml, while others have indicated that 0.2 ng/ml should be the threshold. For most assays, however, truly undetectable levels are at least <0.1 ng/ml. Such differences have led to confusing literature regarding the efficacy of radical surgery and the timing at which adjunctive treatment should be applied.

When there is evidence of failure either of external radiation or radioactive seed implantation, salvage radical prostatectomy has been claimed to have some success. In this setting morbidity (vis-a-vis incontinence and impotence) may be greater. Unfortunately, many instances of radiation failure are accompanied by metastatic disease, and surgical attempts have often led to positive margins and compromised quality of life. Hormonal therapy may be the safest approach in this setting, even though it ultimately may not be curative.

At the time this book is written, the following therapies are still experimental or theoretical in nature, and therefore comparatively little is known about their applicability and effectiveness. More about these matters may be established by the time you are reading this book, so further inquiry is definitely advisable:

⬥ *Suramin drug therapy:* Suramin is an experimental drug now being used in clinical trials to treat prostate cancer patients who prove resistant to hormone therapy—as many as fifty thousand Americans each year. It works by binding to cancer cells and inhibiting their production of "growth factors." Dr. Arie Belldegrun, associate professor of urology at the UCLA School of Medicine and cohead of the suramin trials (along with Dr. Peter Rosen, UCLA professor of hematology/oncology), explains the process as follows:

> Cancer cells secrete nutrients into their environment, then absorb them on their surface; this in

turn enables the cells to develop more rapidly. Suramin disrupts the loop and is a prototype of a new group of agents that operate differently from anything we've ever known before.

Although suramin therapy is not designed to cure the cancer, it shows promise of being a safe and effective way of extending life and reducing pain for patients who otherwise have no options. So far, clinical trials have not shown significant results.

◊ *Hyperthermia:* More commonly associated with treating benign prostate enlargement (BPH), hyperthermia involves using localized heat produced by microwaves to destroy prostate cancer cells. It is administered on an outpatient basis and is easy to tolerate. Currently, it is approved by the FDA for treatment of prostate cancer, but is only being pursued in a very limited number of clinical trials.

◊ *Immunotherapy:* Still in the laboratory stage of development, immunotherapy involves using drugs to improve the performance of the body's natural defense system in identifying and killing prostate cancer cells. A long-range goal among immunotherapists is to develop the capability of making a vaccine from a patient's own body to prevent any recurrence of his prostate cancer.

To date, immunotherapy remains hypothetical. Although numerous experiments with animals do suggest that it is *possibly* effective, clinical studies have never documented any actual effectiveness in treating human cancers.

◊ *Genetic therapy:* It is hoped that eventually new genes can be manufactured and introduced into the body to make:

◊ (a) tissue cells that are more resistant to cancer; and/or

⋄   (b) immune-system cells that are better at fighting cancer.

In general, the approaches towards treatment, stage for
stage, are as follows:

1. "Incidental" stage A1, or T1, disease: This is generally
   diagnosed on pathologic examination of the histologic
   specimen obtained at the time of prostatectomy for symptoms of obstruction in a patient with negative digital rectal examination and probable normal or minimally
   elevated PSA. A policy of surveillance can be elected with
   the risk of progression probably being no greater than
   10–15 percent over the subsequent ten years. For a
   younger patient, surveillance should include periodic PSA
   determination and transrectal ultrasound with biopsy for
   any change that is detected. A change in grade may then
   place the patient in a category for treatment of organ-
   confined disease.

2. "Incidental" stage A1 or T1 high grade (Gleason score >4)
   disease: should be treated as organ-confined disease, with
   the need for treatment other than surveillance because of
   the potential of increased aggressive behavior. For
   patients below the age of sixty-five, radical prostatectomy
   should probably be most strongly considered. For patients
   between ages sixty-five and seventy years, radical prostatectomy or external radiation may be considered. For
   patients above the age of seventy, external radiation
   should be considered rather than radioactive seed implantation because of the difficulty in obtaining good placement of seeds in a patient who has undergone simple
   prostatectomy with variable tissue remnants.

3. Stage T1C disease (no comparable stage according to the
   older classification): The PSA-driven biopsy, which then
   diagnoses the presence of adenocarcinoma, is probably
   the most common means by which prostate cancer is currently diagnosed. Most of these patients have an interme-
   diate Gleason score (5–7) with far fewer having high

scores (8–10) and very few having very low scores (24). Those patients less than 65 years of age are probably best served by radical surgery, even though 30–40 percent of them can be expected to have capsular penetration. Those between ages sixty-five and seventy, or with a limited life expectancy, can be considered for external radiation or radioactive seed implantation. Those above the age of seventy, or those with significant comorbid conditions, might be considered for external radiation, though radioactive seed implantation is still an option. As discussed above, those who have Gleason score 7 or higher have a strong likelihood of having involvement of the seminal vesicles or possible metastatic disease. These are unlikely to achieve cure with any modality. However, if no distant metastatic disease is found, seminal vesicle biopsy should be done. For those with positive biopsies, adjunctive radiation should be considered if brachytherapy is chosen. Generally, preradiation hormonal therapy has appeared to become a standard treatment among radiation oncologists.

4. Stage B1–2 (stage T2a–b): In these patients digital rectal examination has detected the presence of disease. Although considerations in treatment are similar to those outlined for stage T1c above, there is a greater possibility that extension beyond the capsule of the prostate or positive margins will occur with surgery. Therefore, outcome may be worse regardless of what therapy is chosen. The interval of disease-free survival (as defined by the sensitivity of the means by which disease status can be assessed) worsens with increased volume of palpable disease. In these instances care must be taken to define the extent of disease as accurately as possible so as not to apply treatments designed to address stage T2 disease when T3 (stage C) disease is what actually is present.

5. Stage C (T3) adenocarcinom: Patients with this clinical stage of disease are not well served by radical surgery. Unfortunately, the various forms of radiation therapy are also likely to fail. Pretreatment hormonal therapy,

suggested possibly to convert stage C (T3) disease to organ-confined stage B or T2 has not been found to be a realistic expectation.

In these situations treatment is often based on patient demand, and surgery for low volume stage T3 disease or radiation for higher volume disease (preceded by hormonal therapy) is often pursued, but with poor outcome expectation. Many of these patients may already have metastatic disease at diagnosis, and this often becomes manifest within three to five years of initial diagnosis.

7

Considering Alternative Medicine

◊ What alternative medicine is and isn't

◊ Understanding the differences between alternative and complementary medicine

◊ How to think about alternative possibilities

◊ How to question your doctor about alternative medicine

Meet John, Frank, Ed, and Ralph. All four men have been diagnosed with prostate cancer and all have decided to use alternative medicine. Lets look at their choices:

◊ Before his surgery for prostate cancer, John visits a psychologist for lessons in relaxation and healing imagery.

◊ After being diagnosed with early-stage prostate cancer, Frank opts for watchful waiting and begins a series of nutritional changes and herbal supplements while continuing with his routine PSA screenings.

◊ When given the choice of radiation or surgery for his prostate cancer, Ed decides to do neither and begins 714-x treatment with Gaston Naessens in Canada.

◊ Ralph, losing his battle with end-stage prostate cancer, begins treatments that include acupuncture and Traditional Chinese Medicine.

It may surprise you to learn that each of these treatment decisions are all examples of alternative medicine. Nowadays, if you or a loved one has prostate cancer, chances are strong that someone—perhaps several people—will suggest that you try alternative medicine. Consequently, no modern-day book about prostate cancer can be complete without some discussion of this popular recommendation.

In this chapter, you'll learn how to understand the different terms in alternative medicine, discover what questions you should ask alternative practitioners, and understand the importance of communicating with your primary doctor. You'll also develop the thinking skills to evaluate what alternative medicine can and cannot do for you.

What is Alternative Medicine?

Alternative medicine is a broad term that refers to any type of treatment that is not yet accepted by the Western medical establishment as customary. Alternative medicine is often used as a shorthand description to cover both alternative treatments and complementary treatments. Literally, alternative medicine means instead of traditional medicinal treatment. An example would be if you chose to take laetrile instead of having surgery for prostate cancer. Complementary medicine, however, literally means in addition to your tradiitonal treatments. An example would be if you decided to learn relaxation techniques to help you through your surgery for prostate cancer. Sometimes, you will see the more accurate phrase alternative and complementary medicine.

Remember that the term alternative medicine can be confusing. If someone suggests that you use an alternative treatment, you will need to question them further to find out whether the treatment they are referring to is *instead of* or *in addition to* your traditional treatment. Either way, be sure to discuss it with your physician.

You may be surprised to find that you are already using some form of complementary medicine. St. John's Wort, vitamin supplements, echinacea, breathing for relaxation, yoga, and meditation are some of the more popular choices. Usually complementary medicines are compatible with the traditional treatments recommended by your physician.

Let's go back now to the four men discussed at the beginning of this chapter. Notice the different possibilties in their alternative and complementary choices. For example, Ed would be choosing an alternative therapy by taking Naesson treatment in Canada instead of surgery or radiation, while John's choice of relaxation and imagery training would be complementary treatment that enhanced the care of his primary, traditional physician.

How do Men with Prostate Cancer Use Complementary and Alternative Medicines?

First you and your partner need to decide *if* he's going to use alternative and complementary treatments and then you can decide *how* you should use it. There are no formal guidelines or advice on this matter. However, you might consider thinking about these treatments in the following manner:

◊ If you're diagnosed with early stage prostate cancer and come under the category of watchful waiting, you might consider complementary or alternative treatments to boost your immune system while you routinely monitor your medical status.

◊ If you're going to be traditionally treated for prostate cancer, you might explore complementary medicine to manage the side effects of treatment, speed your recovery, enhance your immune system, and lend support for a positive attitude.

◊ If you have late-stage prostate cancer, complementary medicines can be considered to support the ongoing traditional treatment while alternative medicines may offer you additional possibilities if you are told conventional treatments have been exhausted.

(Note that you can find a list of possible choices for prostate cancer by checking the resources at the end of chapter 10. Especially look at the writings of science writer Ralph Moss and physician Dr. Adriane Fugh-Berman.)

In any event, and at all times, consult with your physician and discuss any complementary or alternative treatments that you're considering.

Who Uses Alternative Medicine?

If you're open to considering some form of alternative or complementary medicine, rest assured that you're not alone. According to a 1998 report released by the U.S. government, these treatments are among the fastest growing segments of the U.S. health-care market. In 1990, one-third of the U.S. population used some form of alternative treatment, and predictions are that by the year 2010, at least two-thirds of the U.S. population will have participated in some treatment that's considered to be complementary or alternative medicine.

A Bit of History

It's helpful to understand alternative medicine within an historical context. Traditional Western medicine (the kind you're probably receiving) is actually biomedicine—a chemically and technologically oriented medicine that has a very successful history in finding solutions to bacteria-based infectious disease (for example, the miracle of penicillin).

Although traditional medicine has shown success with certain kinds of cancer, overall it has been far more successful in curing infectious diseases. This limit has led people with cancer and other chronic diseases to search out alternative methods of cure and their search has led to the increasing interest and popularity in both alternative and complementary medicines. Dr. Andrew Weil, noted health physician and trained in both traditional and alternative medicine, has said that blind faith in professional medicine is not healthy. In short, allopathic medicine (traditional medicine) is very good at managing trauma, acute bacterial infections, medical and surgical emergencies, and other crises.

Given this information as background, it is both understandable and reasonable for you to look into alternative or complementary treatments. For prostate cancer patients, the issue is usually a wish to stay in long-term remission (for early-staged prostate cancers), to avoid changes in quality of life, or to find a control or cure for late-stage prostate cancer. Unfortunately, you'll need to exercise extreme caution, particularly if you're considering alternative treatments. The interventions vary from promising to far-fetched, and it will fall to the patients and their family and friends to determine each interverntion's actual value.

One of the reasons this field has been such a landmine is that the old, highly respected interventions that are in standard use in other countries (such as acupuncture) coexist with fly-by-night treatments developed by get-rich-quick entrepreneurs. On the other hand, if you have end-stage prostate cancer and your doctors have done all they can for you, there is little to lose and lots to gain by checking out the various possibilities.

The Office of Alternative Medicine (OAM)/ National Center for Complementary and Alternative Medicine (NCCAM) has grouped alternative and complementary treatments into six different categories for exploration and investigation. These categories are mind/body interventions (such as psychotherapy, support groups, imagery, and prayer), bioelectromagnetics (such as nerve and immune system stimulation), alternative medical systems (such as Traditional Chinese Medicine and Ayervedic), manual treatments (such as osteopathy, chiropractic, or massage), pharmacologic and biological treatments (such as antineoplasms, shark and bovine cartilage, or mistletoe) herbal medicine (such as milk thistle), and diet and nutrition (such as vegetarians or macrobiotics).

Some Unlikely Bedfellows

It may surprise you to learn that any understanding of alternative medicine would be incomplete without an appreciation of politics, science, and economics. Let's take a look at these strange bedfellows as we begin to deepen our understanding of what alternative medicine is and is not.

Politics

Consider the following information:

◊ Acupuncture was recognized in Western medical texts and recommended in the 1892 edition of Sir Willima Osler's *Principles and Practice of Medicine.* This same information, though, was expunged from the editions of this text that were published after his death. Dr. Adriane Fugh-Berman, in her book *Alternative Medicine: What Works* refers to this as postmortem politics.

- The AMA, in its long-standing attempt to squelch chiropractic medicine, voted in 1963 to establish a Committee on Chiropractic which then become the Committee on Quackery. It's primary mission was the containment and ultimate elimination of chiropractic medicine. In 1987 the AMA was found guilty of boycott and conspiracy and subsequently opened the doors to chiropractic medicine. Today, about 85 percent of insurance companies cover chiropractic services.

- Although the medical community has raised a skeptical eyebrow toward herbal medicine, many modern-day miracle drugs have herbal origins. Pain killers such as aspirin (white willow bark), narcotics (opium poppy), capsaicin (chili peppers), and the cancer wonder drugs vincristine and vinblastine (from the periwinkle) and taxol (yew) are a few examples of powerful herbal treatments.

- It's helpful to remember that the current medical recommendations of health promotion through a high fiber diet that reduces the chances of cancer was scorned until the mid-1970s.

- In the 1960s many traditionally trained physicians viewed breast feeding as unnecessary, quirky, and eccentric. Nowadays, breast feeding is the standard recommended practice for new mothers.

As many authorities in alternative medicine note, what's considered to be a fringe treatment today may be a standard treatment within the decade. The line between traditional and alternative, rather than being solid and wide, tends to be fuzzy and narrow and given to frequent change.

Commenting on the politics of medicine, Senator Tom Harkin, one of the primary forces in the formation of the original Center for Alternative Medicine, addressed this political blockade. Science and the government are lagging behind the overwhelming public interest in complementary and alternative health care.

Patients are suffering because of the lack of reliable information available on such practices.

Science

Unfortunately, there are few scientific studies assessing the effectiveness of alternative and complementary medicines. This is a big drawback and makes treatments difficult to evaluate.

When we look for scientific effectiveness, we are looking for the successful outcome of a certain treatment on a large number of individuals in a carefully controlled study. This means that even if you know three men with prostate cancer who were helped with a specific treatment, there may not yet be any proof that this treatment is effective on prostate cancer patients in general.

Unfortunately, many alternatives and complementary treatments are thought to be helpful to some individuals but lack clear proof of effectiveness for larger groups of patients. This is a definite drawback when you're trying to decide if a treatment will work for your partner.

For example, let's say that your partner seriously considering taking shark cartilage as either a complementary or alternative treatment for his advanced prostate cancer. What evidence do you have that this will be helpful? Perhaps you know that your friend Ted was diagnosed with prostate cancer in 1992 and today Ted shows a negligible PSA. He tells you he refused surgery and decided to quit his job, move to the country, give up red meat, and begin taking shark cartilage. He swears that the shark cartilage saved his life.

A scientist's response to Ted's story would be something like the following: It may be true that shark cartilage saved Ted's life, but we have little evidence to prove that this actually happened.

Ted's cure might have been due to the shark cartilage or it could have been due to a change in his diet, to a reduction in stress (quitting his job), to his change in lifestyle (moving to the country), or to all or none of these factors. Ted's cure from prostate cancer could have also been a spontaneous recovery of uncertain and unknown origins; one of those mysterious cases where cancer seems to cure itself. Although Ted attributes his good health to the shark cartilage, we have no way to show that this is actually true. In essence, there is no proof that the shark cartilage was helpful.

To prove the effectiveness of shark cartilage, we would need to run a controlled experiment in which a large number of men with the same stage of prostate cancer were given shark cartilage and compared with another group of men of similar diagnosis who were not given the cartilage, but were given an inactive pill. We would hope to keep all other variables in the men's life under control (like changes in diet, lifestyle, etc.). If the men who took the shark cartilage showed a signifant improvement when compared with the men who did not, then we would have much more confidence in saying that shark cartilage has been proven to be helpful to men with this type of prostate cancer.

Most alternative and complementary treatments have not been subject to this type of rigorous design, so there's often no scientific proof—one way or the other—as to their value.

Economics

Behind the scenes of both traditional and alternative medicines lies the specter of money. Both medicines are billion-dollar businesses, the economics of which heavily impacts the scientific study and availability of treatments.

In particular, many promising alternative treatments have been overlooked because their potential revenues are so limited. Ralph Moss has written extensively about this problem and has emphasized how cancer treatments and research are intertwined with the economics of pharmaceutical companies.

  ◊ The particular patent laws of the United States provide no financial incentive to develop natural methods of treatment, since by definition, these natural methods are not patentable and hence, not profitable. In 1996, Moss estimated that the costs for developing a new drug that complied with FDA regulations would be about $200 million. The only way for a company to recoup this enormous expenditure is through a medicine that they can patent—and monopolize for seventeen years.

◊   The more powerful the treatment, the greater the degree of supervision that's required from highly trained (and expensive) professionals at large, technology oriented (and well-funded) cancer centers. Moss notes that these treatments keep the focus on high-paid cancer specialists and well-funded medical centers. Natural, nontoxic methods, on the other hand, enable primary care healthgivers, or sometimes even the patients themselves and their family members, to administer care.

◊   Alternative treatments, however, are not without their own economic conflicts. No longer a mom-and-pop operation, a recent article in the *New England Journal of Medicine* estimated the out-of-pocket expenditure for alternative medicine to be at $27 billion. Clearly, there's a great incentive in this unregulated industry for unscrupulous salesmen with less than honorable motives.

For many years, science writer Ralph Moss has written about the economic conflicts inherent in cancer treatments. Drug companies are not charities. They exist to serve their employees and stockholders, who invest their money in order to obtain good returns. They incur extraordinary expenses in researching, developing, and marketing new products. Much of this goes to fulfilling the regulatory requirements of the FDA. In return, the government gives them seventeen-year legal monopolies called patents, as a way of recouping these costs.

Points to Consider in Evaluating Alternative and Complementary Treatments

Suggestion One

Generally speaking, an alternative treatment that is used to replace a traditional treatment is medically controversial. It is these treatments that you need to consider most carefully. The pursuit of an alternative treatment may or may not be a reasonable action. One way to think about this is that an alternative treatment may be a reasonable choice when there's little evidence for the success of the mainstream treatment, when mainstream treatments have been exhausted, or in cases where the side effects of mainstream treatments are felt to significantly destroy the quality of your life. Additionally, alternative treatments can be viable choices in cases where the alternative treatment has an equal or better outcome than the traditional treatment.

If you and your partner are considering using an alternative treatment instead of a mainstream treatment, you may be making a major life decision. Your thoughts and rational should be thoroughly discussed with your medical treatment team. Getting second and third opinions about your decision is critical. Explain the logic of why you want to pursue the alternative treatment and then listen carefully to the medical response to see if you have made any errors in thinking.

Marion Morra, associate clinical professor at the Yale School of Nursing, notes that in real life, the cancer physician has probably never met you before and has absolutely no idea of what is going on in your mind. So if you don't share some of your experiences and concerns and ask questions, he or she will never know the best types of treatments to recommend.

Suggestion Two

As in traditional decisions, get at least two to three opinions about the best alternative treatment options.

Remember that medical treatments for prostate cancer do vary, even among traditional physicians. David Bognar, who pursued both alternative and traditional treatments with Cindy, his long-term partner, noted that second opinions are critical. Doctors and pathologists can make mistakes, and competency and accuracy differs from individual to individual and facility to facility. Of patients seeking second opinions at one major cancer center, 70 percent made changes in their treatment. Don't be afraid to ask to have your test results forwarded to another institution or doctor if necessary. Second opinions have become routine, and good doctors are not threatened by them. To help you and your partner with these interviews, consider asking the following questions

- ◊ What are my chances of being cured with the treatment you are suggesting?

- ◊ What are my chances of being cured if I do not use the treatment you are suggesting?

- ◊ What is the chance that I will be alive 5 years from now with this treatment?

- ◊ What is the chance that I will be alive 5 years from now without this treatment?

- ◊ What are the chances that I will have side effects to your treatment? What are these side effects? Are they temporary or permanent?

Suggestion Three

Unless you enjoy rigorous scientific thinking, enlist the help of a friend, co-worker, church volunteer, or relative to help you gather the information; sort through the data and interview the practitioners. If you can't find someone to recruit for this job, consider hiring a university student (in medicine, psychology, research etc.) and paying them an hourly rate to help you with this task. Be sure that the student is familiar with statistics and is able to and comfortable with accessing the Internet and executing a computer search.

Suggestion Four

If the survival odds are in your favor with traditional treatment, your partner may still want to include complementary treatments to help him avoid recurrences and give him an extra advantage. Generally speaking, a truly complementary treatment is one that you and your physician have discussed, that's nontoxic, and that adds a dimension to traditional treatment. Some examples of such treatments are some forms of vitamin therapy, massage therapy, music therapy, aromatherapy, dietary enhancement, meditation, psychotherapy, stress management, visualizations, support groups, and acupuncture. If you're considering a complementary treatment, your job will be somewhat easier than if you considering an alternative treatment, since you'll encounter less resistance from your physician and will be adding on to your treatment instead of choosing between treatments. Most complementary treatments are welcomed by traditional physicians because they can be used to enhance standard medical treatment. Again, complementary treatments have an impact on the body and so they must be discussed with your primary physician.

Suggestion Five

The whole question of alternative and complementary treatments can spark major controversy in your relationship with your partner. Perhaps you believe that such a treatment can be a lifesaver and your partner thinks it's all foolish stuff. Or perhaps your partner is open to these different interventions and you find yourself thinking of these choices as hocus-pocus. For many couples, conversations in this area are fraught with controversy, particularly for interventions that have no clear effectiveness data one way or another.

If this is the case, it will probably be helpful for a partner to ultimately be positive and supportive about the patient's choice of treatment. In the case of nontoxic complementary treatments, we urge even skeptical partners to be supportive from the onset. It may help partners to know that a positive belief in a nontoxic treatment may turn out to be quite helpful for both fighting illness and mobilizing the immune system. Indeed, a study on optimistic beliefs showed that they were linked to higher levels of immune functioning. Consider using our decision-making grid in chapter 6 to help clarify your position on this topic.

Being supportive is usually more difficult if the patient is making an alternative choice that his partner does not agree with. Generally speaking, we recommend that partners tell the patient their honest opinion, state why they believe it to be true, encourage the patient to go for second and third professional opinions, and then back off and support his choice—for ultimately, it is his body, his life, and his decision

Suggestion Six

Be a smart medical consumer. Stay open to new information and remember that doctors cannot know everything. Be suspicious of any treatment that sounds too good to be true. Be suspicious of a traditionally trained physician that rejects all alternative medicines without inquiry. Question any alternative practitioner that denigrates all traditional treatment methods.

Good doctors are open-minded and encourage you to participate in your treatment and accept the fact that each patient is different and no one school of treatment has all the answers for everyone. As Dr. Andrew Weil, nutritional expert, has noted "The first guidelines I can give you is that there is no one right way. A particular diet may be right for you at this stage of your life, but it may not be right for me, and it may not be right for you a year from now. We are all different physically and biochemically, with different and changing dietary needs" (Weil 1995, 3). It is this willingness to see people as individuals, and to shun a one-size-fits-all approach, that is the hallmark of good practitioners—both traditional and alternative.

Even though you know you should ask for a second and third opinion, some patients are uncomfortable doing so and "worried" about hurting their physician's feelings. Marion Morra suggests a script to solve this problem. If you are the patient or the partner and are uncomfortable with this issue, try saying "I don't really want to go for a second opinion, but I want one for my wife's (or daughter's or friend's) peace of mind." It's a white lie that might save your life.

Don't Forget the Power of Mental Medicine

Mental medicine or mind/body medicine is a way of accessing your mind to help heal your body. Mental medicine includes psychotherapy, support groups, imagery, relaxation, meditation, and other forms of mental or psychological activity. Recently, the power of mental medicine has gained increasing recognition and support among traditional healers.

One type of mental medicine that often occurs in scientific experiments is a placebo. The placebo, or placebo effect as it is usually called, occurs when a person's belief is activated to help them get better. A placebo can be anything that the patient believes willl help them, whether it's an inactive pill or loving care or simple attention. Overall the average effect of the placebo is an astounding 33 percent—far more effective than some well-respected drug treatments.

David Bognar in documenting his experiences with alternative medicine, notes:

During the past thirty years, the growing body of research indicating connections between our minds and our bodies has shattered the long-held belief in Western medicine that these two systems were separate. The evidence is clear. The mind can have an effect on the quality of life and even on the course of an illness.

Noted health guru Dr. Andrew Weil states:

> For many years immunologists maintained that the immune system was the only autonomous system of the body, the only one that operated free of external controls. This is a silly idea—no system of the body is autonomous. All are interconnected especially with the nervous system ... clearly emotional states like grief and depression can interfere with immunity just as loving can enhance it. You do not need to know anymore than that to be motivated to improve your emotional health ... Do not try to stop or fight a negative mental state. Instead, put energy into creating a positive state and the negative will tend to resolve.

One of the most positive benefits of pursuing complementary treatments, even in the absence of clear effectiveness data, is that if an approach makes you feel like you are doing something to help yourself, then you are probably are helping yourself. We have clear evidence that optimism and hope affects health and immunity.

Let's say that John has decided to eliminate red meat, begin yoga classes, and join a prostate cancer support group. Most alternative and traditional practitioners would applaud John's decision for two reasons. First, there's some evidence that each of these changes promotes health, enhances immunity, and increases the sense of well-being. Secondly, we know that John's enthusiasm and belief in these choices and sense of control over his health and life will, in itself, promote a level of increased health. Doctor Andrew Weil, commenting on the power of mental medicine, notes that part of the reason for success (of alternative diets) is the mental shift represented by the decision to follow a demanding nutritional program. That mental shift may be more important than the specifics of a program.

Seconding the importance of mental beliefs and attitude, noted cancer cell biologist and licensed psychologist Joan Borysenko observes:

> It is remarkable to me that any of us could have forgotten that we have one body-mind and not a mind and a

body. Who is there who hasn't had a really embarrassing thought and then instantly blushed and recognized— of course, I have one body-mind! A thought or emotion causes my entire vasculature system to change, my entire hormonal profile to change. Now we know that's true. Our very thoughts and opinions affect the hormonal profile in our blood. They affect our heart rate and may affect our immune system.

What a powerful wonderful drug to have in your personal medicine cabinet. Of all the complementary and alternative possibilities, mental medicine may be most powerful one that has ever existed! Many of the suggestions in "Dr. Barbara and Dr. Sandy's Take Care Tips" (chapter 8) are truly mental medicine. So are the relaxation and visualization exercises in the same chapter.

As you can see, the field of alternative and complementary medicine is intricate and complicated. The available data and research is a complex intertwine of politics, science, and economics that effect the available data and research. Reaching a decision is far from simple. The best you can do is be an open-minded, knowledgeable, and skeptical consumer, contributing actively to decisions about your treatment.

8

Living through the Treatment Process

◊ Putting practical affairs in order

◊ Dealing with family, friends, and the medical team

◊ Maintaining a healthy lifestyle

◊ What to expect regarding specific therapies

◊ Handling fear, loneliness, and emotional exhaustion

Dr. Elisabeth Kübler-Ross, a world-famous authority on how patients and their partners cope with life-threatening illnesses, once described the treatment period for cancer as "living under the darkest of shadows." Referring to this period, she said,

"People are like stained-glass windows. They sparkle and shine when the sun is out, but when the darkness sets in, their true beauty is revealed only if there is a light from within."

Undergoing treatment for prostate cancer, whatever specific form that treatment may take, challenges both the patient and his primary caregiver to make their own way through a strange, inscrutable new life: day by day, hour by hour, minute by minute. As they do, they discover that their own inner strengths begin to shine through, helping to illuminate the path. The more effectively these strengths can be tapped and drawn upon, the brighter, clearer, and more reassuringly negotiable the path will be.

This chapter is designed to help you and your partner cope as best you can with the practical and emotional issues that commonly arise *during* the treatment process, from the moment you've made your treatment choice, until after the treatment has run its course (which, in some cases involving hormone therapy or chemotherapy, may constitute the rest of the patient's life). During this "shadow period," you can comfort yourselves to a certain degree by relying on your doctor, but there are likely to be many times when you'll feel physically and emotionally exhausted. Whether or not it's medically necessary to act as swiftly as possible (usually it's not), most people who cope with cancer do feel a *psychological* need to act swiftly. Plus, it takes a great deal of sheer effort on your part to make treatment arrangements, cooperate with treatment procedures, and retailor your "normal" life to accommodate treatment demands. Meanwhile, concern about the posttreatment future never goes away, nor does the need for you to make decisions that no one else can make.

The treatment period is a time that brings out the worst as well as the best in your partner and you. As much as you can, you want it to be the best! With that in mind, we'll be using this chapter to explore four different aspects of shining through the treatment process:

- ◆ *general guidelines* for handling practical issues, whatever the specific treatment may be, such as putting legal and business affairs in order, dealing with family and friends, maintaining a healthy diet and lifestyle, and consulting with members of the medical team;

◊ what to expect regarding *specific therapies*—typical procedures as well as possible complications for each of the major treatments, including surgery, radiation, hormone therapy, and chemotherapy;

◊ handling different types of *emotional issues* that commonly arise for patients and caregivers during the treatment period, including anxiety attacks, loneliness, and emotional exhaustion.

Let's begin by looking at general guidelines.

General Guidelines

1. Putting Your Faith and Trust in Your Physician.

Once your partner and you have made the decision to proceed with treatment under a particular physician's direction, it's important to *commit* yourself to that decision. This means allowing the physician to employ his or her knowledge and skill with your full cooperation and support.

Your decision to proceed with the treatment carries with it the assumption that you have already given your doctor your personal "seal of approval." In other words, through some sort of predecision qualifying process (hopefully using many of the guidelines offered in chapter 4 of this book), you and the patient have determined for yourselves that your doctor is capable, knowledgeable, compassionate, and understanding. Therefore, it's in your best interests to follow his or her instructions to the letter and, if you consult with other doctors or practice other therapies, to make sure that he knows.

In the event that a reasonable cause arises for questioning the doctor's judgment, competence, or concern, the patient (and, ideally, you as well) should be sure to discuss the matter with him or her—or, if available, a relatively neutral medical authority, such as a patient representative (or similarly designated person) on the staff of the doctor's hospital—before taking steps to change doctors. After all, you once approved of the doctor you are now questioning, and it's possible that your faith in this doctor can be restored fairly easily: for example, by clearing up a simple misunderstanding or by agreeing mutually to a different and better way of managing the treatment process. Reconciliation, if possible, is often the best solution to a crisis in confidence.

When a shift in doctors *does* seem advisable even after your partner and you have tried your best to resolve matters, don't be afraid to speak up, and don't feel that you have to be either sweetly apologetic or defiantly aggressive. Instead, adopt a straightforward and business-like manner. The doctor you are leaving should be prepared and willing to cooperate. Remember that this type of shift in medical care is not uncommon: patients change doctors, and doctors refer patients to other doctors, for all sorts of reasons, and there are more or less standard procedures to ease the process. Above all, try to remain civil and communicative with the doctor you are leaving. However tense, awkward, or even hostile the situation may be, remember that your goal is to arrange a smooth, effective, and therapeutic transition from one physician's care to another.

2. Remember that the Patient is Never Without Power and Rights During the Course of Treatment.

Throughout the treatment process, the patient always retains his decision-making prerogative. Your partner and/or you should never be afraid to ask questions of your doctor or any other member of the medical team or to insist upon timely, sufficient, and comprehensible answers.

Always keep in mind that the *patient*, and not simply the *cancer*, should be the focus of treatment. Anytime that you and your partner feel left out, confused, doubtful, overridden, or simply overwhelmed, you are perfectly entitled to step in and make sure that this all important focus is maintained and honored. It is just as vital, if not more so, for members of the medical team to under-stand you, as it is for you to understand *them*.

3. Putting Practical Affairs in Order.

If you are the primary caregiver for your partner, you are the captain of his support system and the one most likely to bear the burden for what he does *not* do. Therefore, prior to the treatment process itself, consider suggesting to your partner that he put his personal affairs in order and supply you with all the relevant documentation as soon as he reasonably can. Ideally, he should do all of the following things that are relevant, not so much because he may die but more because it will make life easier for him, you, and other people around you during the course of this highly unpredictable illness:

◊ Your partner should complete a "living will" and a "durable power of attorney." These documents help ensure that he will receive the type and extent of medical and life-support care that he wants, even if he is physically incapable of communicating his desires (e.g., unconscious, in a coma, or medicated to the point that he cannot reason effectively).

To cover the latter situations, each of the above-mentioned documents designates a "health-care agent" or "health-care proxy" who can act on his behalf by enforcing his preferences, either as they are stated in the documents themselves or as the agent/proxy understands or interprets them. The agent/proxy can be you, the primary caregiver, or anyone else who is close to the patient and easily contactable. Alternate agents or proxies can also be designated.

Forms for both documents are available from your state or provincial Department of Health. Your partner can complete them without the help of a lawyer; however, in order to make sure that there are no misunderstandings, he (and/or you) may want to consult with your doctor about any specific life-threatening or life-supporting medical treatments that he may face in the course of his illness, so that these treatments can be listed individually, along with his specific wishes regarding them. Also, the documents will need the signatures of one or two witnesses who are *not* designated as agents/proxies.

The terms of these documents differ from state to state and are applicable *only* within the state that issues them. Therefore, depending on the circumstances, your partner may need to fill out forms from more than one state: for example, if he is going out of state for treatment, or if he will be spending an extended vacation—or regular weekend getaways—in another state anytime during or after the treatment process.

◊   If your partner has been handling the household bills and finances, ask him to do so as much in advance as he can, and to leave clearly written instructions for you or someone else on how to continue managing these matters. The same strategy applies to household and automobile maintenance tasks.

◊   It would help if your partner made one annotated phone-and-address list of all the key people in his life—relatives, friends, lawyers, accountants, insurance representatives, doctors, therapists, coworkers, et cetera—so that you *and* others can easily use it if and when necessary. It may be a good idea to make copies of this list and give them in advance to major members of your support team, who, in an emergency, may have to act quickly in your behalf.

◊   Ask your partner to make sure that his last will and testament is up to date. Ideally, he should also make one annotated list for you (and, if necessary, others) of all his major financial assets and how they can be accessed.

♦ If your partner is employed, he should consider discussing his treatment plans with his boss, supervisor, staff, and all important colleagues. If he thinks that this is feasible, then in a "two-way" conversation, he should explain clearly and concisely what the situation is, communicate what support he expects, and find out how he can best work in advance to prepare others for an indefinite leave of absence and/or period of reduced work time on his part.

He should also consider talking with the person in charge of his company's health-care benefits to find out exactly what coverage is available, how to expedite claims processing, and when to expect bill payment. If appropriate, all of this information should then be communicated to you—even the talks with his boss, supervisor, staff, and important colleagues, at least in summary fashion. (NOTE: The Rehabilitation Act of 1973, a federal law, prohibits employer discrimination against cancer patients. So do laws in many states.)

4. Closely Monitor Each Step of the Treatment.

It's generally much easier to cope with the known than the unknown, and the sheer activity of keeping informed about things can be emotionally stabilizing for a patient *and* his caregiver in a time of crisis. Ask for a full explanation of, and rationale for, each treatment procedure in advance, and then do what background research you can, right away, to become more knowledgeable about it.

If the patient agrees and it's suitable for the particular treatment involved, you or someone else close to the patient should accompany or wait for him whenever treatment is administered exercising moral support and keeping an eye, an ear and, if needed, a mouth alert for anything unusual that might happen. After each treatment procedure, either the patient, you, or the designated support person should ask the doctor for a full report, and question the doctor and anyone else on the medical team to make sure that you understand what you are told.

On any of the occasions when you meet with the doctor, remember to take notes and/or to audiotape the conversation. You may also want to bring a trusted and supportive family member or friend along, preferably a major member of your support team, not only to ensure that you remember everything the doctor says but also to offer "sounding-board" counsel and solace after the meeting. In addition, the person you bring with you will become better acquainted with your doctor (which could turn out to be very helpful), more informed about your partner's situation, and all the more committed to helping you monitor it.

5. Keep Your Support Team Informed, and Assign Appropriate Responsibilities as Necessary.

All during the course of treatment, regularly update key members of your support team (or, if you don't have a functioning "team"—as described in chapter 5—your closest friends and family members) about your partner's progress. Preferably, this update should occur on a prearranged and dependable basis, such as every Sunday evening and/or the day after every major treatment procedure. You can then use these "updates" as occasions to ask for help on specific tasks: e.g., providing car trips to the clinic, doing some last-minute shopping that you can't do, tracking down medical information that you'd like to have, or sitting with the patient when you won't be able to do so.

To avoid the potentially burdensome task of having to make numerous "update" phone calls on a regular basis, you may want to appoint one person as a "relay" person—someone who can pass along your personal report to all the other key people, and who is available for calls from these key people when you're not (or whenever they don't feel comfortable disturbing you). An updated outgoing message on an answering machine can also make this job easier. You may also want to empower this relay person as your principal deputy, supplying him/her with copies of all the major data and documents relating to your partner's illness and business/household affairs, so that he or she can take over from you at a moment's notice whenever necessary. Just make sure that everyone on your support team realizes and accepts this person's deputy status.

6. Work to Make Visits Between the Patient and any Well-wishers as Pleasant and Comfortable as Possible for Everyone Involved.

With your partner's consent (as much as possible), mediate tactfully between your partner and his visitors so that you can arrange in advance for get-togethers that will be enjoyable and not too taxing on either party. For all visits, the physical and emotional welfare of your partner should be your main concern.

Once the visit is taking place, try as much as possible to let your partner speak for himself, since he is the main focus of the visit and may derive a great deal of benefit from "rousing" himself to attend to others. Certainly resist any temptation to say things to him during the visit like "Now, don't be so crabby" or "You're real glad Mark came, aren't you?" Taking up a conversational lull can be helpful (even though there's nothing wrong with a lull in itself), but directing your partner's behavior or putting words into his mouth—however well meaning—can be very annoying or embarrassing to him, especially during this period of unusually high emotional stress.

Many caregivers are sorely—and, often, understandably—tempted to use the presence of a visitor as an opportunity to reinforce a message that the patient may be resisting ("I keep telling him he shouldn't get up and down so much"), or to voice a complaint about the patient that still rankles ("He never lets anyone know how he really feels"). Regardless of the truth of what you have to say, a visit is *not* an appropriate occasion to speak out. It puts your already weakened partner on the defensive, just when he wants to make as good an impression as he can, and it puts the visitor in the awkward position of having to take sides.

Do what you can to help ensure that visits are well timed to occur when your partner is not too tired or occupied with other tasks like eating, napping, taking care of personal affairs, or undergoing some therapeutic procedure. Typically, a person's daily energy level is best an hour or two before midday lunch and an hour or two before dinner, but you should watch closely to determine your partner's personal energy cycles. If visits are taking place during a hospital stay, everyone should try to respect hospital visiting hours and visitors-at-a-time limits, because they are designed to help guarantee that the patient's energies won't be too challenged.

Visits should also be appropriate in length—usually no more than twenty minutes to a half hour at a stretch, although sometimes the patient may welcome or expect a longer visit, especially if he is comfortably ensconced at home. You and your partner may want to agree upon some distinct, unmistakable, and yet unobtrusive signal that you can give to each other in the visitor's presence when either of you wants to terminate the visit soon—like saying "By the way, we must not forget to call the doctor later," or rubbing the right side of the nose.

For comfort's sake, you and the patient may want to discuss ahead of time the best possible setting, routine, and accoutrements for the particular visit at hand. For example, if two or three people are making a bedside visit at the same time, you will want to pre-arrange chairs and lighting so that no one winds up enduring an awkward position in silence. If young children are coming along with the adult visitors, you may want to set up some child-related activity at another location so that the children can entertain themselves without disturbing the patient.

It might be nice to enhance a bedroom visiting locale with new art objects, fresh flowers, better lights, and more convenient chairs and side tables. Your partner may feel more upbeat and presentable during visits if he has especially attractive and comfortable new lounging outfits: robes, slippers, loose-fitting trousers, and pullover shirts and sweaters that suit his style and current mobility.

An excellent general rule for managing successful visits is to let all potential visitors know the best visiting procedures long before they arrive—procedures that you and your partner have agreed upon ahead of time. Don't be afraid to initiate conversations with people about the best times to come by, the most appropriate length of time for them to stay, and, if necessary, how you would recommend that the visit take place. Everyone involved, including the visitor, can benefit from, and appreciate, this type of thoughtful planning.

7. Be Especially Careful to Eat, Sleep, Exercise, and Conduct Daily Activities in a Healthy Manner.

At no time is it more important for people to protect, preserve, and enhance their overall physical well-being than when they are going through periods of unusual physical and emotional stress. Cancer patients are all the healthier—and happier—for being healthy in general. In medical terminology, they have "better functional status," which can enhance their chances of survival. And their partners, too, feel better and more capable if they respect their body's need for *extra* care and attention during this exceptionally stressful period.

The rewards of such care and attention are multidimensional and can be realized almost immediately. One of the caregivers interviewed for this book remarked:

> At first [during the postdiagnosis and treatment period], my husband and I must have unconsciously decided that nothing else mattered, healthwise, but the treatment itself. We continually ate whatever we liked, or, in my case, whatever was at hand, and we abandoned our daily walks. I, personally, was only sleeping four or five hours a night, so I didn't have the energy to do any better. It seemed right for us not to worry about "normal" health habits because my husband was too preoccupied with his cancer and I had my hands full just running around managing one crisis after another.
>
> Then, a friend got me to start taking better care of myself and my husband by giving higher priority to

normal, healthy patterns in everyday life: healthy meals, healthy exercise, healthy sleep. After just a week of making sure we followed a healthier daily routine, ignoring some of our crisis-management impulses, our stamina and our spirits picked up dramatically. Things in general no longer seemed as tense or depressing.

This testimony reminds us, once again, that the patient as a whole—and not the illness all by itself—should be the primary focus throughout the treatment process for prostate cancer or any other major disease. During this period, when some very serious health-related developments are beyond one's direct control, it's usually both physically and psychologically beneficial for the patient and his partner to assume control of whatever health-related matters they can.

For more specific advice, especially relating to the patient's particular lifestyle and treatment protocol, be sure to talk with your doctor.

Healthy Eating

These tips for the patient are based on expert recommendations for good nutrition in general. They do not necessarily evolve from scientific research relating to prostate cancer in particular, although much of that research supports them. Anyone can benefit from following them, including you, the all-important caregiver!

◊ Maintain a low-fat diet by limiting your intake of red meat (no more than once a week), dairy products (except nonfat), eggs, butter, and saturated oils (in most vegetable oils, which can be replaced with healthier, polyunsaturated oils like olive, peanut, sunflower, or canola).

◊ Restrict your daily consumption of caffeine and alcohol. A patient on medication may have to abstain from these substances. Try to eliminate tobacco consumption altogether.

◊ Avoid foods with a lot of chemical additives (check labels).

◊ Eat a lot of high-fiber foods, such as cereals, whole-grain breads, dark beans, broccoli, cabbage, and Brussels sprouts.

◊ Eat a lot of foods high in beta-carotene or vitamins A, C, and E (all "antioxidants," which assist healthy cell growth): fresh fruits (especially apricots and cantaloupes); green, leafy vegetables (especially Brussels sprouts, spinach, and cabbage); carrots (especially fresh); and whole grains.

◊ If the treatment—or treatment-related anxiety—tends to cause nausea, indigestion, vomiting, or loss of appetite, avoid eating right before or after treatment. During the day, eat several small meals as hunger arises, rather than one or two big meals at a set time. Eat slowly, chew well, and avoid mealtime distractions like reading or watching TV. Cut out spicy or sweet food in favor of blander items like bread, chicken, cereal, and sherbet. If the problem persists, ask your doctor about possible medications.

◊ In the event of diarrhea, eat smaller amounts of food at each sitting, and temporarily avoid foods that produce gas such as dark beans and, regrettably, other high-fiber foods). Drink clear liquids (water and broths) to clean your bowels, and increase your intake of potassium (especially abundant in bananas and potatoes). Don't take antidiarrhea medication without first consulting your doctor.

◊ If constipated, eat smaller amounts of food at each sitting. Increase your intake of water and high-fiber foods like cereals and fresh fruits, but in *modest* amounts, or you may trigger diarrhea. Don't take anticonstipation medication without first consulting your doctor.

Healthy Exercise

With a health crisis imposing so many demands on your time and energy, you and your partner may decide to forego any physical exercise routines. It's an understandable but lamentable response. For both of you, regular physical exercise can be particularly beneficial at this time, helping your body work more efficiently, relieving your emotional stress, improving your self-esteem and "body image," and, best of all. making you feel better all over! Here are some tips for staying in shape.

◊ The patient should be sure to consult with the doctor before planning or undertaking any program of regular exercise. It would also be wise for you, the caregiver, to do the same.

◊ Begin with modest goals and a gentle program for *daily* exercise. Remember that your main objective is to exercise regularly and faithfully. You don't want to set up a program so difficult or unpleasant that you wind up abandoning it after a few days. A bedridden patient who can't do aerobic exercises may still be able to do easy stretches and isometrics, as well as lift small hand or wrist weights.

◊ With the help of qualified advice (available from doctors, many books and videos, and some health club personnel), design a program that includes different types of activities: *stretching* exercises to increase flexibility, *aerobic* exercises to build up energy and endurance (like walking), and *muscle building* exercises to improve strength and tone (like isometrics, sit-ups, or weight lifting).

◊ Incorporate exercise into your daily schedule as comfortably and conveniently as you can. You can do all three types of exercise during the same half hour or hour each day, or you can do each segment at a different time: for example, stretching in the morning, calisthenics in the late afternoon, and an after-dinner walk. It's easier to maintain an exercise program if you do the same things each day at the same time, but don't hesitate to vary the schedule on days when it's more convenient to do so.

◊ Make exercising as pleasant as possible. Wear suitable and attractive clothing especially designed for exercise. Create a compelling environment for at-home exercises: for example, a corner of the bedroom that's free of clutter and decorated with pictures that inspire perseverance. Choose a time and a place for walks that will provide the most enjoyment.

◊ If possible and desirable, you and your partner should try to exercise together. It not only helps each of you to maintain your program (and watch out for any overdoing on the other person's part), but also enables you to spend more time together when you're not so preoccupied with the illness or other pressing matters.

◊ Besides doing regular exercises, take advantage of exercise opportunities that arise spontaneously: walking instead of driving the car, climbing stairs instead of taking the elevator, gardening for a half hour instead of watching TV, et cetera.

8. Keep in Mind that Unexpected Developments Can Arise at Any Time.

During the treatment period, it's best to take one day at a time. Tomorrow can always present you with a new scenario—one that frustrates, prolongs, intensifies, or renews the treatment period. For example:

◊ Surgery, a new round of testing, or a suddenly emerging symptom may reveal that your partner's cancer is more advanced than originally diagnosed, which may dictate more of the same kind of treatment, perhaps in a stronger or more far-reaching form, or a different treatment altogether.

◊ A treatment may result in unanticipated complications or side effects: an allergic rash from a medication, unusually severe fatigue after chemotherapy, a heart attack during surgery.

◊ You may suddenly find out that your partner has to go out of town for treatment. In fact, both of you may have to establish temporary residence out of town for several weeks, in order to allow for sufficient treatment plus recuperation.

◊ Even after you've been led to believe that the treatment has been successful, that the treatment period is over, and that your troubles are behind you, there is always the prospect of recurrence. You may think that your partner's cancer has been completely removed, halted, or cast into remission, only to find out weeks, months, or years later that cancer is spreading once again in his body.

No matter what unexpected development may occur, remember that nothing is to be gained by dreading the future, and everything is to be gained by being realistic. Throughout the treatment period and for several years afterward, think of yourself as "on call" to do what you *reasonably* can from one day to another, and keep yourself *reasonably* informed about the range of possibilities—negative as well as positive—relating to your partner's condition and treatment. Try to avoid willfully refusing to face the fact that anything might happen. Instead, be open minded as well as optimistic.

Specific Therapies: What to Expect

Each case of prostate cancer is unique, depending upon the man's age, physical condition, psychological character, lifestyle, and overall support system. And individual treatment procedures in general vary widely, according to the specific patient, doctor, technology, and hospital or other medical facility involved.

For these reasons, as well as the fact that treatment advances are being made at such a rapid rate these days, it's impossible to provide in these pages a reliable step-by-step description of each major treatment process that your particular man may encounter. Indeed, it would be irresponsible to attempt to do so. Your doctor should be the source for any specific information regarding your man's treatment and the possible consequences.

However, the following discussion offers a *general* picture— circa 1995—of typical procedures as well as possible complications for each of the major treatments. These treatments include surgery, radiation, hormone therapy, and chemotherapy. For additional information, see chapter 6, "Choosing among Treatment Options." For a discussion of problems, treatments, and coping strategies associated specifically with posttreatment incontinence and impotence, see chapter 9, "After Treatment: Sex, Continence, and Peace of Mind."

Surgery

After hospitalization on the day of surgery or the night before, patients may or may not be given an enema for cleansing followed by a sterilizing solution known as a "bowel prep." The latter mixture of antibiotics can help prevent an infection just in case the rectum is penetrated during surgery (a possible complication that rarely causes significant problems).

The surgery itself, as described in chapter 6, is a major operation lasting around three hours, beginning with the removal and inspection of the pelvic lymph nodes to make sure the cancer hasn't spread (assuming this removal hasn't been done previously), and proceeding to the removal of the entire prostate gland. If cancerous cells are found in the lymph nodes, it is likely that the prostate itself will not be removed. Instead, the surgery will be concluded and a different, more systemic course of treatment will be planned, usually involving hormone treatment.

The patient coming out of surgery is taken into the hospital's intensive care unit, where he regains consciousness—usually within an hour. He will probably be uncomfortable, but it's not likely to be seriously painful. He'll have a Foley catheter running through his penis and up to the bladder and, usually, two or three so-called "drains" in the lower abdomen: small openings to the surface that serve as outlets for any loose blood or urine from the body interior.

Because the patient's normal intestinal contractions will be temporarily slowed down as a result of the operation, there *may* be a tube running through his nose into his stomach, through which excess intestinal fluids can be sucked out by machine. Generally, this tube isn't considered necessary; but if it is installed as a precaution, he will not be able to eat normally until it is removed (usually in three or four days, by which time the drains have also been removed). The catheter stays in place for two to three weeks: not only to prevent urine leakage, but also to serve as a splint for the healing of the ureter.

In some cases, the patient will also be supplied with a patient-administered analgesic pump (more commonly known as a PCA pump), which allows him to manage his own medications for discomfort. This small, noncumbersome device will stay implanted in the patient's body for as long a time as is deemed necessary by the doctor and the patient.

Caregivers of prostatectomy patients often speak of how disconcerting it is to visit the patient immediately after surgery. A forty-year-old woman interviewed for this book remarked:

> Seeing [my husband] for the first time after the surgery, when he was wheeled from the intensive care unit to his room, was the biggest shock of the whole illness. His face was swollen, his legs were all wrapped up in inflatable gadgets, and he seemed bandaged from the waist down. I expected grogginess, but he was totally out of it. He looked and acted deathly. The doctors said they were pleased, but I couldn't help being scared. In fact, he recovered very well.

In most cases, the postsurgical patient shows rapid improvement. He can sit up and take short walks along hospital hallways as early as twenty-four hours after surgery. There will be a certain amount of added discomfort associated with these movements, but it's generally minor and more than offset by the joy of regaining mobility. Discomfort associated with the postoperative healing process as a whole may require prescribed medications for a number of days.

On the average, a postprostatectomy patient stays in the hospital around five to seven days (although this time period varies considerably from patient to patient and doctor to doctor), and the catheter is later removed on an outpatient basis. Following the removal of the catheter, the patient usually doesn't regain continence for several days, and there may well be recurring incidents of incontinence for weeks or even months afterward, necessitating the ongoing use of pads. Full recovery, if it's going to happen, should take place within a year.

As for sex involving penetration or male climax, it may be anywhere from four months to a year before the patient can achieve and sustain erections (the physical healing itself takes around two months). If the patient is still not able to do so a year after surgery, it is very likely that nerve damage—a frequently unavoidable consequence of surgery—has rendered him permanently impotent. For more information on coping with impotence, loss of sexual desire, and other sexual dysfunctions, see chapter 9.

Radiation Therapy

External radiation therapy (the most common form of radiation therapy) typically takes six weeks to two months, involving multiple treatments each week at a clinic or hospital outpatient department. It begins with an X-ray session that establishes the "target point" for the radiation beam. This point is marked on the patient's body by a strong, cleansing-resistant dye that should remain visible throughout the treatment period. If it starts to fade, call this fact to the attention of your medical team; do *not* try to "color" it yourself.

The external radiation treatments themselves are painless, similar in feeling to a normal X-ray procedure. However, they sometimes have unpleasant aspects. In a 1994 interview for *The New York Times Magazine*, Michael Milken, the billionaire financier who served prison time for securities fraud and went on to found the Association for the Cure of Cancer of the Prostate (Cap Cure), found his external radiation treatments uncomfortable:

> In order to hold you in the proper position during radiation they have to create molds of you. I've got my tushy mold at home. At the hospital sometimes I would be lying down in an uncomfortable position for an hour and a half. I would then actually meditate on the radiation table.

Furthermore, the aftereffects of radiation therapy can be very distressing. As the treatment progresses, with the cancer-killing rays causing more and more damage to healthy as well as unhealthy tissue, the patient may become more and more susceptible to fatigue, diarrhea, and/or frequent and painful urination. Some patients experience one or more of these symptoms for only a few hours after treatment, and then only mildly. Others suffer several of these symptoms on an ongoing basis, occasionally quite severely.

If and when your man has any of these symptoms, ask a member of your medical team for suggestions on how to ease any pain and discomfort: specific strategies work differently for different patients. For general tips on how to cope with fatigue—and with the radiation patient's increased risk of infection—see the discussion of these topics under "Chemotherapy" later in this chapter.

An external radiation patient is often troubled to some degree by dry or irritated skin in the area of treatment. As a general rule, it's a good idea to expose this skin to the air (but not the sun) as much as possible and to touch it as little as possible, which means avoiding clothes that rub it. Do not take it upon yourself to apply any creams, lotions, or cold packs to the area without first checking with your doctor.

External radiation patients can suffer temporary impotence and incontinence up to six months after the last treatment. In some cases, impotence or incontinence is a permanent aftereffect of treatment. The likelihood of either condition is less for radiation therapy patients than it is for surgery patients.

Internal radiation therapy (appropriate only for early stage prostate cancers) often requires an initial hospital stay of several days, during which the radioactive materials are implanted in the prostate gland and allowed to do their most active work. The implantation procedure is a minor operation (a needle is inserted through the perineum), but the following few days can greatly tax the patient's overall energy level. For this reason, he may not be able to handle visitors—at least for more than ten or twenty minutes at a stretch.

In about 30 percent of internal radiation therapy cases, the implantation is performed on an outpatient basis rather than during a hospital stay. Doctors choose this course of action for their patients either because the level of radioactivity is relatively low, compared to other cases, and therefore less likely to cause seriously adverse side effects, or because the overall health of the patient robust enough to tolerate possible side effects with only outpatient treatment as a backup.

After receiving the implants, the patient usually does not need any further treatments. After a few months of ever-diminishing activity, the implants will cease to emit any radioactivity, and hopefully the early-stage cancer will have been halted or destroyed. On the whole, internal radiation therapy involves fewer and less intense side effects than external radiation therapy. It does not cause any irritation to the skin itself and has a much lower incidence of permanent impotence or incontinence.

Hormone Therapy

Protocols for drug-based hormone therapy vary considerably from patient to patient, according to the specific drug used, the dosage involved, the precise nature and extent of the cancer, and the patient's overall health. Treatment may involve daily, weekly, or monthly pills and/or injections. The patient (and/or his caregiver) may be able to self-administer the treatment at home, or it may have to be administered in a clinic, hospital outpatient department, or doctor's office. The entire therapy can last weeks, months, or even years. Frequently, it is administered in conjunction with radiation therapy, thereby adding further variables.

Thus, living through drug-based hormone therapy means paying particularly close attention to side effects and seeking frequent updates from your doctor about what to expect given the progress so far. It also requires making an especially strong effort not to get discouraged—either by the many emotional and physical ups and downs that tend to accompany the treatment period, or by the many unknowns and ambiguities that make the treatment process itself unpredictable.

As mentioned in chapter 6, hormone therapy involving LH-RH agonists or estrogen commonly results in a loss of sexual desire, impotence (often, but not necessarily, permanent), and hot flashes (up to two or three times a day). Other possible side effects are stomach and intestinal problems, including loss of appetite, nausea, diarrhea, and vomiting.

The hot flashes and stomach/intestinal problems can sometimes be treated fairly effectively with medications, so discuss such symptoms with your doctor as soon as they appear. Above all, support your partner in getting proper daily nutrition. Not only is it important for his general health and for the success of the therapy, but it can also help minimize the occurrence or impact of negative side effects. If your partner is unable, unwilling, or disinclined to eat "normally," work out an acceptable solution with your doctor.

Hormone therapy involving castration (orchiectomy) may or may not require a short hospital stay. The surgery itself is not complicated, nor is there much time, pain, discomfort, or lack of mobility associated with recovery. After surgery, the patient almost always experiences a loss of sexual appetite and permanent impotence. In many cases, he also feels occasional hot flashes. He does not, however, suffer any treatment-related stomach or intestinal problems.

Chemotherapy

Like drug-based hormone therapy, chemotherapy takes a wide variety of forms, depending mainly on the patient's age and general health as well as on the nature and spread of the cancer. Doctors and their patients can choose among many different types of drugs and treatment methods (e.g., pills or injections; in-hospital, out-patient, or at-home administration), with individual cases sometimes involving unexpected, midcourse shifts in protocol. The overall length and frequency of treatment is usually very difficult to project: too much hangs upon how things go for the patient week by week and month by month.

The drugs used in chemotherapy have their strongest destructive effect on the body's fastest-growing cells. Besides the cancerous cells that are the primary target of the therapy, these fastest-growing cells include hair-follicle cells, the cells in the gastrointestinal lining, the infection-fighting white cells in the bloodstream, and the blood-clotting platelets in the bloodstream. As a result, men undergoing chemotherapy tend to experience hair loss, gastrointestinal problems (such as poor appetite, nausea, or vomiting), a lower resistance to infections (e.g., sores, colds, and flu), and an increased tendency to bleed or bruise.

These latter two side effects—a lower resistance to infection and an increased tendency to bleed or bruise can be especially troublesome. Here are some tips for avoiding or managing them:

Guarding against Infection and Bleeding

◊ You, your partner, and anyone else who has regular, intimate contact with your partner should wash their hands with soap frequently during the day to remove possible infectious agents. This is especially advisable before eating and after using the toilet. Also, make sure to shower or bathe daily.

◊ As much as possible, your partner should avoid all activities that could result in bleeding: for example, flossing or vigorous toothbrushing (check alternatives with your dentist), shaving with a razor (switch to an electric shaver), engaging in "rough"

games or exercise, using hand-tools without wearing gloves, blowing his nose hard, or walking
barefoot.

◊ It's not advisable for your partner to take any
medications—prescription or over-the-counter without first checking with his doctor. Some medical
compounds like aspirin, tend to impair the bloodstream's clotting abilities.

◊ It is advisable for your partner to report any cuts,
scrapes, sores, or symptoms of infection (such as
fever, chills, coughing, sneezing, unusual sweating,
differences in urination) to a member of his medical
team, so that he can obtain the best advice for
prompt treatment.

Another side effect that is common during chemotherapy is
fatigue, which can range unpredictably and intermittently from
vague listlessness to complete physical exhaustion. Here are some
guidelines for keeping fatigue-related problems to a minimum:

Guarding against Fatigue

◊ The patient should monitor, in writing his daily
energy levels—keeping track of when lowpoints
occur, how long they last, and how, specifically, he
feels during them. From time to time (under normal
circumstances, every week to ten days), he should
review these levels with his doctor, who may know
ways of ameliorating certain fatigue problems (for
example, by medication or blood transfusion).

◊ He should limit his daily activities to a comfortable
level, avoiding events or activities that require extra
energy. It helps to make daily to-do lists, underscor-
ing those items that are the most important and
making sure to do them first. It also helps to dele-
gate certain activities to other people who are willing and able to perform them.

- He should make a special effort to move slowly and surely at all times, but especially when exercising, lifting things, or getting in or out of cars, chairs, or bed.

- He should build more regular "sleep-time" or "rest-time" into his daily schedule: perhaps an early afternoon nap, an hour of quiet reading after dinner, an earlier-than-usual bedtime, and/or a later-than-usual rising in the morning.

- He should be sure to maintain a healthy diet and to engage in regular (but *moderate*) exercise.

- He should cease movement and rest the minute he feels any unusual tiredness or light-headedness.

- He should tell his doctor or a member of his medical team about any pain he is experiencing *as soon as possible*. He should not wait until it gets worse, since pain is usually easier to control when it's mild rather than strong.

- He should bear in mind that doctors tend to be conservative in prescribing pain control measures. This means that he should not hesitate to speak up if and when he feels pain, even if he is already being treated for pain. He should not feel that he's being a bad patient by complaining, nor should he assume that everything's already being done to manage the pain that can—or should—be done.

- He should not worry about becoming addicted to pain medications—one of the most common, and ungrounded, fears among cancer patients. Almost always, the medication can be reduced gradually as the pain wanes, thereby preventing addiction. Remember, patients in pain *need* pain relief; it isn't just a treat to get them high.

- He should not take any pain medications on his own without first consulting the doctor. Even the

Controlling Pain

Compared to many other types of cancer, prostate cancer does not usually cause much pain unless it is very far advanced, nor is there much pain associated with the major treatments for prostate cancer (except as side effects of intensive radiation or chemotherapy). Nevertheless, pain is always a possibility where cancer or medicaltreatment is concerned; and when pain strikes, there are things a man can and should do about it to ensure optimum health and quality of life. The bottom line is, pain can be controlled, and there's no reason for him not to exercise as much control over it as he can.

◊ He should keep good track of his pain, so that he can describe it accurately to his doctor or a member of his medical team. This means doing the best he can to answer the following questions:

  ◊ Where is it, precisely?

  ◊ What does it feel like? Is it sharp, dull, throbbing, steady, burning, tingling, gnawing? Use your imagination to find the right words or metaphors.

  ◊ How bad is it on a scale of 1 to 10 (10 being the worst)? If there are recurring attacks of the same kind of pain, do they vary in intensity? How so, using the scale? Does the pain ever interfere with your ability to concentrate, sleep, eat, perform normal activities? How so?

  ◊ What seems to make you feel better or worse when you have the pain? Heat? Cold? Lying down? Distraction?

⬥ How does any prescribed treatment for the pain seem to be working? Does it cut the pain in half? Does it cease to work after an hour? Does it upset your stomach?

⬥ Has the pain changed in any way over time? Grown stronger or weaker? Progressed from achy to tingly?

most common over-the-counter pain relievers, like aspirin or ibuprofen, can produce undesirable side effects due to the illness or the already-existing treatment protocol.

⬥ He should take any pain medications *as prescribed*. Deciding on his own to skip a dose (for example, because he isn't feeling pain at that particular time) or to double up on a dose (for example, because the pain seems especially strong) can seriously undermine the medication's ongoing effectiveness.

⬥ He should keep good records of his prescribed pain medications, noting the name, dosage, time period, and any reactions—positive or negative. These records can be invaluable in conversations with his doctor, members of his medical team, other doctors, or other health professionals.

⬥ He should make sure to have enough pain medication on hand by getting his prescriptions refilled four or five days *before* his supply is due to run out.

⬥ He should talk to his doctor or a member of his medical team about the possible effectiveness of nondrug-related methods for relieving his pain. These methods include biofeedback; breathing and relaxation techniques; massage, pressure, and vibration; transcutaneous electrical nerve stimulation (TENS); exercise; distraction (e.g., listening to

music); hot or cold packs; immobilization and bed
rest.

◊   He should ask his doctor or a member of his medical team about the possible effectiveness of pain
support groups or short-term psychotherapy aimed
at dealing with pain. He should obtain the government's "Cancer Pain Guideline" by calling
1-800-4-CANCER (or 1-800-422-6237).

Emotional Issues

When patients *and* their caregivers talk about the treatment period
for prostate cancer, regardless of what form that treatment may
take, they most often complain about three different types of emotional problems: (1) fear, (2) loneliness, and (3) emotional exhaustion, or what is known in the military world as "battle fatigue."
Each of these problems manifests itself differently in the patient as
opposed to his caregiver; but, typically, the caregiver is left to deal
with *both* problems.

Fear

Fear is a common and natural response to any situation that
is novel, uncertain, and/or capable of producing negative results.
Being treated for prostate cancer—or standing by a loved one
while he is treated for prostate cancer—certainly qualifies as this
type of situation! You're worried about treatment-related discomfort, pain, disfigurement, disability, and death. You're concerned
about the temporary disruption of your "normal" life, and just
how long that disruption may be. You fret about money, schedul-
ing, and the performance of daily tasks. You agonize over the
future—now, suddenly, a terrifying mystery.

It is unreasonable to think that you or your partner can or
should get rid of fear entirely. In fact, fear is not an altogether
negative emotion. It can alert you to needs, "discharge" feelings of
depression or despair, and even mobilize you to take positive
actions. Instead of simply trying to ignore, deny, or avoid fear, try

learning to recognize it for what it is, to face it squarely, and to keep it under control.

Many people fall to realize that they are suffering from fear until it is well advanced and therefore far more difficult to control. Sometimes, you or your partner may feel fear *physically* rather than *emotionally.* Your symptoms may include any one or more of the following:

◊ an inability to relax, characterized by restlessness, sleeplessness, the "fidgets," or problems in concentrating or remembering

◊ persistent shallow breathing, perhaps even difficulty in breathing deeply when you deliberately try to do so

◊ muscular "shakiness" (try holding your hand still, with fingers spread)

◊ upset stomach, for no other apparent reason

◊ rapid heartbeat, for no other apparent reason

◊ light-headedness or sweating, for no other apparent reason

The most extreme physical expression of fear is the panic attack, which can strike without any warning and last for several minutes to an hour. The person suffering a panic attack feels as if he or she has definitely lost control. Besides palpitations, a rapid heartbeat, and/or very intense forms of several of the symptoms already mentioned, he or she also experiences acute psychological distress—a feeling of going insane, of having a heart attack, of dying, or of facing certain disaster. Part of the "panic" for the sufferer is not knowing why the attack is happening: it seems much too sudden, too strong, and too weird to be caused by any specific fears one might harbor. This only goes to show that fear is a much more potent force than we normally realize. Again, fear is not something to be dismissed, ridiculed, underestimated, or overindulged.

How, then, can a cancer patient and his partner best deal with the various fears that they may encounter during the treatment process? The best approach is a three-part strategy: identification, education, and relaxation.

"Identifying" your fear means saying to yourself, as soon as you realize it, "I am experiencing fear." Then, you need to go on to determine what, precisely, is causing the fear; for example, "I'm afraid that the surgery tomorrow won't go well," or "I'm scared by the way my partner looks at me," or "I'm worried that I'll have trouble running all my errands today." If you don't take this identification step, your vague, unlabeled fear can expand to include all the fears you're capable of having. Thus, the treatment-related fear turns into a much larger anxiety about being incompetent, unsafe, and unhappy in general.

The next step, education, involves looking at your fear more objectively and answering questions like:

◊ *Why am I having this fear right now?* There may be factors contributing to your fear besides the obvious ones; for example, a fear about an impending operation may be aggravated by the fact that you're tired, that you're remembering a bad experience that you once had with an operation, that you're also worried about a late mortgage payment, or that you're not sure what you'll actually be doing during the day of the operation.

◊ *What can I do to help alleviate the cause of this particular fear?* For example, the more informed you are about the procedures involved in an upcoming operation, the less likely you are to let your imagination run wild with a false, nightmarish scenario. Assuming that you're troubled by the memory of a past operation, you can make a special effort to pinpoint how the upcoming operation is intrinsically different and less threatening. It may also be helpful to think of intense fears as being like an iceberg. When we look at an iceberg, we are actually seeing the top 10 percent; the most massive part of the iceberg lies below the surface.

When we are very afraid, a small part of that

fear, let's say 10 percent, is based in reality, and it is quite normal and healthy to experience some fear or anxiety during an illness. But when we are very afraid, or terrified, or panicky, we find that 90 percent of the fear is based on an underlying exaggeration or a "catastrophization" of the problem.

It helps to remember that when fears get out of hand, the reality of danger is usually much smaller than our greatest fears.

◊ *What can I do to temper the effects of this particular fear?* For example, if you tend to awaken in the middle of the night with fear and can't get back to sleep, you can research and practice ways to handle sleeplessness. Maybe you can solve the problem by reciting a special poem to yourself, or getting up for a while to read, or taking a mild medication, or changing the way you go to bed.

Finally, you and your partner need to learn ways to incorporate more relaxation into your day-to-day life, especially during those times when you are most beset by fear. Simply put, relaxation in this context means literally resting and seeking peace, not doing something active or looking for stimulation.

Besides lying down, taking naps, or rocking back and forth on a porch swing, you might try a specific visualization technique for achieving a more tranquil, less fearful state of mind. To perform a visualization, you assume a comfortable position (preferably lying down), close your eyes, and create a particular scenario with your "mind's eye"—one that you can dwell within, imaginatively, for several minutes at a time (anywhere from one to twenty minutes, depending on your skill and the circumstances). You can use the visualization model below, or you can search for other models among the many visualization books or audiotapes in the "self-help" market (just be sure to look for models specifically designed to induce relaxation). You might also ask your doctor, a member of your medical team, or your therapist for suggestions.

Visualization for Relaxing Fears

1. Take several deep breaths to relax your body physically. Meanwhile, empty your mind of all thoughts and worries.

2. Let the word *peace* fill your mind. Repeating it slowly in your mind, imagine yourself entering into a natural environment that is very peaceful, comforting, and safe to you. It may be a place that exists—or used to exist—in the real world: a corner of a garden in back of your home, a beach you once visited on a vacation, or a field where you used to daydream as a child. Or it may be a place you simply make up for this exercise, such as a magical woodland clearing or a beautiful desert landscape similar to one you saw in a movie.

3. Allow yourself to relax in this environment, imaginatively experiencing it with *all* of your senses: the soothing sights, sounds, fragrances, textures, and temperatures.

4. Imagine that the sun, shining down softly upon you, gradually warms and calms your body, infusing you with a sense of peace and well-being. Imagine yourself becoming more and more still and secure.

5. Imagine that a new, refreshed "you" slowly, gracefully, and pleasurably emerges from your body, like a butterfly from a cocoon. This "new you" is you at your best, strongest, most confident, and most hopeful.

6. Keep this image of the new you before you for a while, as it wanders about your special place. Admire its resplendent beauty and power.

7. Imagine this new you reentering your body as you slowly repeat the word *peace*. Keep repeating the word *peace* as you gradually bring yourself back to the "real" world and open your eyes.

The more you practice a particular visualization, the better it gets. Just trust your mind to create and enjoy whatever it will. If you find your mind wandering away from the visualization as you're performing it, don't be concerned. Just take a deep breath and gently lead your mind back.

You may want to help yourself become more proficient with a visualization by setting aside one or more *regular* times each day to perform it. In addition, you can go ahead and use it *spontaneously* whenever you become particularly fearful and need immediate relaxation.

Loneliness

The words of the patients and caregivers interviewed for this book speak eloquently of the loneliness that each partner can experience during the course of prostate cancer treatment:

> I felt as if I'd somehow accidentally been transported to some other planet, and that no one around me could possibly understand, much less appreciate, what I was going through.
>
> —a sixty-five-year-old patient

> I went from being part of a couple to being less than a single person. It was like being a kid who's lost. I wanted to cry out for help, for attention, for someone to take care of me. But as an adult, and especially as an adult having to be strong in a crisis, I just couldn't let myself do that.
>
> —a sixty-year-old wife of a patient

> All day long [taking care of my father at his house], I'd look forward to the nighttime, when I could go home and be by myself. But then when I finally was able to be alone, I'd find that I couldn't take it. Time after time, I'd get scared, or depressed, or angry. I'd call friends, desperate to talk or to do something, but they had their own lives and couldn't get away that easily.
>
> —a forty-five-year-old daughter of a patient

It's solitary confinement, being a cancer patient, even if
you have a crowd of people swirling around you. You
can't help but feel cut off, cast away, abandoned,
unwanted, and unwantable.

—a sixty-one-year-old patient

In chapter 4, we discussed that the best way to avoid or cope
with loneliness throughout the illness is for each of you— patient
and caregiver—to establish, in advance, one close friend or family
member who will serve as your primary, first-resort source of
companionship, comfort, and camaraderie. This should be a person with whom you can easily be intimate: someone who knows
you well, who is good at sharing and keeping confidences, who is
dependable, and, most important, who tends to make you feel
better. If you or your partner did not set up this kind of "buddy"
relationship *before* the treatment process began, it's not too late to
do so after the treatment has started.

Once you've determined whom you would like to assume
this role (ideally, each of you will have your own buddy), talk
with this person about your possible needs, and then ask whether
he or she would be willing to "be there" for you if and when you
had those needs. You don't have to conduct a long, involved conversation. For example, you could say, "It would be a great help
to me to have someone I can talk with, or have fun with, when
things get too overwhelming. Would you be this person for me?"

Choose a time to have this talk when you are fairly com-
posed and can discuss your situation calmly, allowing the other
person to respond as he or she wishes without feeling unduly
pressured. This is much more polite and effective than waiting
until a "crisis" of loneliness forces you to call someone and
demand his or her attention right away.

Other options for avoiding or combating loneliness include
joining a patient and/or partner support group (ask your doctor
for suggestions) or seeking short-term therapy. Many hospitals
offer professionally led group counseling for people dealing with
cancer and/or any serious illness. Often, you can participate in
these groups for as long a time—or as short a time—as you wish.
Some groups are open not only to patients and their caregivers

but also to family members and other special people in the patient's life. Different groups offer different kinds of interactions. Some use music, poetry, art, or role playing to help members explore their feelings together; others are "mentor" oriented, with veteran patients or caretakers helping those who are newly facing the same problems.

Aside from group counseling, you might consider family counseling or individual therapy. Remember that it's vitally important to have *someone* to whom you can communicate your feelings and to whom you can turn in a crisis when you're under the extreme pressures of coping with a life-threatening illness. Medical doctors, hospital social workers, or hospital psychologists are good sources for referral to psychologists, psychiatrists, or other mental health professionals who are trained specifically to counsel people affected by serious illness.

Emotional Exhaustion

Inevitably there will be times during the treatment process when you or your man are simply tired of it all. Your emotional energies are drained, and you feel the death-in-life, bone-weariness, or complete emptiness that soldiers call "battle fatigue."

It's easy to understand and appreciate how *patients* get into this state: They're the ones who are actually being treated for illness, who are holding center stage in all the drama of treatment, and who are most directly and poignantly confronting death. What is often misunderstood, unappreciated, and therefore overlooked is how *caregivers* become emotionally exhausted. As a caregiver yourself, you need to be extra aware of the reasons why caregivers come to suffer burnout. These reasons include:

◊ being overworked, literally, by having to perform more tasks than usual, day after day, many of them new and/or uncomfortable;

◊ having to make decisions in very uncertain circumstances;

◊   taking on personal responsibility for the patient's well-being: both consciously and subconsciously;

◊   feeling therapeutically powerless to affect the course of the illness;

◊   overidentifying not only with the patient, but also with close friends and family members who are affected by the illness;

◊   facing a newly threatening and unknowable future, as well as one's own mortality.

The more aware you are of the causes for becoming emotionally exhausted, the more you can work toward alleviating those causes. For example, the minute you suspect that you might be working too much, you can begin enlisting help or letting certain low-priority things slide. If you hear yourself complaining to a friend about how powerless you are to help your partner, you can take it as a warning signal that you are definitely being too hard on yourself.

The antidote to emotional exhaustion is to do something that's emotionally restorative. For practical, timetested suggestions, see "Dr. Barbara and Dr. Sandy's Take-Care Tips," below.

Dr. Barbara and Dr. Sandy's Take-Care Tips

Going through the experience of prostate cancer demands a great deal of the patient *and* the caregiver, emotionally as well as physically. While you're traveling on this journey, you need "filling" stations along the way to replenish yourselves. Anything that takes you out of your day-to-day routine can be restorative. It doesn't have to be a week at an expensive spa. Here are some more practical ideas:

1. Make a "goody contract" with yourself. Literally write a list of specific ways that you can treat yourself, and

then commit to giving yourself at least one of these "goodies" a week.

2. Tune in to parts of your body that are feeling tense and do something specific to relieve that tension. ask a friend or family member to give you a rubdown, or get a professional massage. If you can't do this, consider an especially long, hot, luxurious bath or an equally long, hot, luxurious shower—preferably at a time of day when you rarely have one, so it's a treat rather than part of a routine.

3. Try a class in aquafitness or aquaerobics. It can be very soothing to play in the water, with upbeat music, among other people who are smiling and enjoying themselves.

4. Sign up for a course in yoga or tai chi. Both of these gentle-movement practices teach deep relaxation and valuable stress-survival skills.

5. Rent a silly all-laughs movie, make some popcorn, and tune out the world!

6. Go for a quiet walk alone or with a good friend.

7. Eat something outrageous! Try an item from the "exotic foods" aisle of your supermarket or a "comfort food" from your childhood that you haven't had for years. You might even assemble a weird banquet-for-two (you and your partner) of all your favorite foods. Set a truly fantastical table or have a free-style picnic on the floor. Celebrate absolutely nothing but the fact that you and your partner are alive at this particular moment!

8. If anyone volunteers to do something, let them do it! If a casual acquaintance suggests doing your laundry, say "Yes!"

9. Hug yourself.

10. Have a good cry.

11. Make a list of all the helpful things you did this week for other people, and then reread the list and thank yourself.

12. Read a novel that you've always been meaning to read but never have. Or reread a beloved novel you haven't read for a long time.

13. Daydream, remembering that you can't be punished for even the wildest fantasies!

14. Watch clouds sail across the sky.

15. Dance around your living room, with or without recorded music.

16. Sing for yourself. Make it a concert!

17. When the rain falls, brew a cup of herbal tea and drink it where you can listen undisturbed by anything else. Think of all the times in your life when rain was a gentle visitor.

18. Close your eyes, focus on your breathing, and repeat to yourself "the grass grows all by itself."

19. Avoid the negative. Disengage yourself, at least temporarily, from the things that are emotionally toxic in your environment: unpleasant noises, a messy room, a nagging telephone, a dreaded task, a looming crisis, a "friend" who always brings you down.

20. Focus on the positive. Ask yourself, *What was the high point of the past week for me? How, or why, did I have that expenence? Is there anything I can do to have that experience—or a similar one—again?*

21. Remind yourself that you are entitled to be cared for and to enjoy life, even under these circumstances!

22. Find something, anything at all, to give thanks for.

9

After Treatment:
Sex, Continence,
and Peace of Mind

⬥ Coping with impotence and other sex-related
  problems

⬥ Choosing and enjoying artificial procedures and
  devices for achieving erection

⬥ Managing and overcoming incontinence

⬥ Dealing with uncertainty and depression

A properly managed convalescence after treatment is vitally
important to a patient recovering from any serious illness, but it is
even more critical to a patient recovering from prostate cancer.
Seldom discussed and often willfully ignored, the psychological

pressures that men feel immediately after prostate cancer treatment are uniquely strong and difficult to endure.

After treatment, men who have had prostate cancer exist, on some level, in a state of perpetual trauma: not just about whether they're going to live or die, now that science has done what it can, but also about whether they're going to live as "men" or as "babies." Are they going to be able to perform well sexually and to urinate in a natural, manly manner? Or are they going to be reduced to the status of infants, with no sex and little or no control over their bladders? How will the outcome influence their desire to live? How will it affect their relationship with their partner?

Most of us try to avoid thinking about our health as much as we can. It's in our human nature not to go looking for trouble but rather to hide from it or ignore it. We seldom pay attention to our bodily functions until they present us with life-interfering problems that we simply can't ignore. Then, our attention becomes acute, and we grow thoroughly bewildered. In our strange new state of confusion and near-panic, we can't rely on our own judgment about the seriousness of our situation. We wonder how much of the physical trouble we're experiencing is, in fact, brand new, and how much has been intermittent or slowly developing for years and years, without our really noticing it. Being so hypersensitive, how can we assess what feels "normal" and what doesn't, and whether we're getting better or worse, or staying just the same?

In the aftermath of treatment for prostate cancer, these questions bedevil the patient's mind—and therefore the caregiver's mind—about sexuality and urination in general, especially if the patient is experiencing "unusual" difficulties, but even if he is not. Given the life-threatening, mind-bending crisis that has intervened between his previous daily life and his present one, how can he or his caregiver make sensible, reassuring assessments about how his physical state of being *now* compares with his physical state of being *before*? Any sexual or urinary problem he encounters in his posttreatment life is bound to provoke more concern than a similar problem did (or would have done) in his pretreatment life.

Adding to the confusion is the fact that posttreatment patients are naturally inclined to compare their physical condition with that of other patients who have had similar treatments—people whom they actually know, or hear about from their doctors and friends, or see on television, or read about in books and magazines. They also can't help but judge their posttreatment state in terms of how close—or how far—it is from the "best case" scenario that was projected before treatment. Thus they open themselves up to feeling like failures, to harboring unrealistic expectations, or to abandoning hope unnecessarily.

The most effective means of resolving all these emotional dilemmas is for both the patient and the caregiver to live in the present, not in the past, and to resist the tendency to compare the patient's condition with anyone else's condition. Each person's problems—and solutions—are unique, depending not only on the specific nature of the illness and its treatment but also on countless other variables, including the patient's overall physical well-being, his personality, his lifestyle, his relationships, and all the circumstances that surround his daily life. In making their way through this highly unpredictable posttreatment period, the patient and his caregiver need to think of it as a card game: You can't do anything about the hand that you're dealt, but you certainly can, and should, learn to play a poor hand well.

In this chapter, we will look first at posttreatment problems and solutions related to the patient's sexuality. Then we'll consider issues related to his continence and, finally, issues related to the patient's—and the caregiver's—general peace of mind.

Sex, Manhood, and Sensuality

(For more specific information about the risks of impotence related to specific treatments, see chapters 6 and 8.)

Without a doubt the biggest sex-related fear that men have, whether or not they are posttreatment prostate cancer patients, is "Will I be able to get an erection?" It is difficult for women to appreciate just how significant—and legitimate—this concern is for a man. Due to biological, as well as other, more behaviorally conditioned, reasons, a man's capacity for experiencing sexual pleasure is strongly focused upon his ability to achieve an erection that can lead to orgasm. And even in the healthiest, most well-rested, and most sexually eager of men, this ability is not just physiological—a basic arousal response—but, to a certain extent, psychological as well. It is easily affected by the man's underlying mental or emotional state at the time and by the current quality of his relationship with his sexual partner.

Naturally, a man who has been treated for prostate cancer is especially susceptible to worrying about his ability to have an erection. If he's had a prostatectomy, he does, in fact, run a relatively high risk of being permanently impotent afterward—that is, of never being able to achieve a satisfyingly rigid erection by natural means. Again, the reasons could be physical (surgery-related damage to the nerves facilitating erection), psychological (emotional trauma that interferes with sexual arousal), or both. Assuming he doesn't become permanently impotent, he is virtually sure to go through a temporary postoperative period of persistent or intermittent impotence. Other treatments, including radiation, also involve a risk of permanent impotency. But regardless of the specific treatment involved, *any* prostate cancer patient is likely to experience greater-than-normal anxiety about his ability to have an erection, if only because he's been compelled to spend so much time and energy worrying about how healthy he really is "down there."

What about Fertility?

Male *fertility*—the ability to father a child due to the continued production of healthy sperm—is not to be confused with male *potency*—the ability to have an erection leading to orgasm. A man can be fertile and yet impotent (the net effect of which may or may not result in his being able to father a child), or potent and yet infertile.

Although some men remain fertile well into their seventies, the fertility of most men has begun steadily declining by the time they reach age fifty, when prostate cancer starts becoming a possible issue. Because of this natural decline, as well as the fact that most men prefer not to become fathers after age fifty, prostate cancer patients are usually not concerned about loss of fertility due to cancer or its treatment. Fertile men facing treatment who want to ensure that they can still father a child after treatment are advised to provide sperm samples for lab refrigeration *before* treatment, so that their partner can—possibly—be artificially impregnated at a later date.

Medical hormone therapy and chemotherapy (depending on the specific treatment protocol) commonly do render a previously fertile man infertile. Surgical hormone treatment, i.e., castration, definitely results in infertility. In most cases, so does a prostatectomy, although not necessarily. Sometimes, in the case of a simple (as opposed to a radical) prostatectomy, postoperative infertility is due primarily to retrograde ejaculation: the sperm that previously was ejected through the penis is now ejected "backward" into the bladder. In this situation, there are two alternatives for recapturing the sperm: (1) a doctor can use a catheter to draw the sperm from the bladder; or (2) the patient can urinate *immediately* after ejaculation into a container, and then take the container to a medical lab to have the sperm filtered out of the urine.

Impotence, however, is only one of three broad sex-related issues that can trouble a man who has undergone—or who is undergoing—treatment for prostate cancer. A second issue involves his general sense of *manhood*, or, in other words, his gender identity: how virile and masterful will he feel after having become a highly dependent "victim" of prostate cancer, and how will he redefine his masculinity if he no longer has the same capabilities to perform sexually or even to urinate? Finally, there is the issue of a man's overall *sensuality*. Now that he's been forced to associate his body so closely with illness and decay, discomfort and distress, how can he recapture a sense of physical wholeness and aliveness? And, assuming he has new difficulties performing sexually in the manner to which he and his partner have grown accustomed, how can he learn to enjoy and share his physical feelings in other ways, perhaps in ways that he has never even tried before? Let's look at each of these three issues separately.

Impotence

(NOTE: In the context of sexual performance—and of the possible side effects of prostate cancer and its treatments—the word *impotence* refers to the inability to achieve an erection. It does *not* refer to the inability to have an orgasm, for which an erection is not physically necessary (although it may well be *psychologically* necessary, depending on the individual). In other contexts, the word *impotence* has the more general meaning of "powerlessness." For this reason, doctors and mental health professionals who are referring to sex-related impotence often prefer the more accurate, if more awkward, expression *erectile dysfunction* to *impotence*. Nevertheless, the word *impotence* is retained throughout this book because it is far more commonly used.)

Many posttreatment prostate cancer patients fail to realize that they may be dealing with "normal" impotency difficulties instead of—or at the same time that they're experiencing—illness- or treatment-related impotence difficulties. Impotence is a much greater problem among men over age forty in general than is commonly acknowledged.

According to a 1994 federally financed study conducted by the New England Research Institute (the largest study of its kind since the Kinsey report), over half of American men over age forty experience impotence to some degree. The frequency steadily increases with age. Among forty-year-old men in the study, 5 percent described themselves as totally impotent; another 15 percent, moderately impotent; and another 15 percent, minimally impotent. Among men age seventy, the corresponding figures were 15 percent totally, 32 percent moderately, and 20 percent minimally.

The factors leading to "normal" age-related impotence tend to be multiple in each individual case. Almost always there is an accompanying lack of sexual desire that may be a cause, or an effect, or some combination of both. Possible physical causes are vascular difficulties (such as clogged arteries or high blood pressure, which can impede the flow of blood to the penis); the use of prescription or recreational drugs (including alcohol and, in some cases, nicotine); fatigue; illness (almost any kind that entails serious pain or loss of energy, but especially illnesses related to the pelvis, spinal cord, or endrocine system); injury to the groin; or, possibly, a decline in hormone levels associated with a natural stage in a man's life that is now being called "male menopause" or "viropause" (see chapter 1 for more discussion of this stage). The most common psychological causes of impotence are situational stress, depression, anger, and low self-esteem. In diagnosing any case of impotence, including impotence experienced by a posttreatment prostate cancer patient, all of these factors, both physical and psychological, must be investigated.

If your partner believes that his posttreatment impotence problems may only be temporary, encourage him to consult his doctor and a qualified psychotherapist or sexologist to determine the best way of coping with those problems. It may be very helpful for you to accompany your partner on these consultations, depending on how each of you feels and what the doctor or therapist recommends. Or, if your partner prefers to go alone, or resists the idea altogether, you might consider going to a doctor or a therapist on your own behalf, that is, to determine how you can best deal with your personal problems associated with your partner's impotence.

Meanwhile, be especially understanding and responsive toward your partner. If appropriate and desirable, try to encourage him to participate in other forms of sexual or erotic expression that don't require an erection, such as those mentioned below in "Beyond the Erection."

Alternatively, if medical and psychological experts have given you and your partner every reason to believe that the impotence is

---

Beyond the Erection

Here are twenty-five wonderful ways that you and your partner can experience sexual and sensual pleasure without the need for an erection:

1. hugging

2. kissing

3. cuddling

4. cradling

5. rubbing

6. massaging (especially with oils)

7. stroking (try slowly, with a feather)

8. fondling

9. tonguing

10. licking (perhaps adding to your pleasure with choco-
    late sauce, apple butter, whipped cream, or brandy)

11. sucking

12. performing male-to-female oral sex

13. performing male-to-female manual stimulation

14. playing with sex toys (such as vibrators; restraints;
    and vacuum, friction, or massage devices)

15. experimenting with techniques described in sex
    manuals

16. wrestling

17. watching erotic movies together

18. reading erotic stories to each other

19. painting each other's body (ask for body paints at art
    supply shops) or try some chocolate body paint!

20. bathing or showering together

21. sharing sexual fantasies

22. frolicking naked or near naked in a secluded outdoor
    spot

23. dancing very close and seductively

24. role-playing favorite seduction scenarios (strangers
    sharing a train compartment, movie star and servant—
    use your imagination)

25. lounging in sensuous undergarments in an especially
    sensuous environment (satin sheets, candlelight. soft
    music or an "ocean" sound-effects tape—again, use
    your imagination)

permanent, and if both of you still want to enjoy sexual activities that involve an erect penis, there are three main options that a man has for artificially inducing an erection: using a vacuum pump, self-injecting a drug, or having a penile implant (a mechanical device—or prosthesis—surgically placed inside the penis).

For those individuals who have undergone radical prostatectomy that has resulted in erectile dysfunction, the use of Viagra may permit recovery of erectile function in 20 percent of cases. Many men, however, become concerned about the potential side effects of Viagra and choose not to employ this potential option. In many instances, the degree of erection is not sufficient to permit vaginal penetration. Greater success is often achieved by intracavernosal injection of vasoactive agents.

On first consideration, the idea of relying on an artificial procedure or device to induce an erection is sure to seem alien and repellent to most men; and the first few attempts at sex with any new procedure or device are bound to feel clumsy (as are most first attempts at sex of any kind). But if a patient and his partner persevere through this initial awkward period, they're very likely to discover that such reliance is easier, more effective, and more natural than they had imagined.

A sensitive doctor or therapist can be an enormous help in coaching a man—or, ideally, a couple—through the "start-up" phase. So can a prostate cancer support group, as revealed in the following account offered by a sixty-five-year-old spouse of a prostate cancer patient who became impotent as a result of his prostatectomy:

> When we told the surgeon about the impotence, he said, "It could be in your head," which, true or not, only terrified us. First we had the worry about the cancer, then the operation, and now this sexual problem! The surgeon said very calmly, "Well, we have a prosthesis," which, again, it just didn't help to hear.
>
> As for me, I was scared silly, because we'd had sexual problems before. As for him, he was in denial. He'd go around seeming happy. He tried porno movies and reported that he did get some sensation. He tried to masturbate. But basically he was resigned. He couldn't

bring himself to ask for the prosthesis. He felt *This is my fate.* He wouldn't even talk seriously about a prosthesis for six or seven months after surgery, and the doctors just kept telling me, "Give him time." But I was devastated about this.

Finally, after we went to see a sex therapist, he got the prosthesis and seemed to be enjoying it, but he was not achieving orgasm, so sex just gradually slipped away. He avoided it. Then, last summer at an Us Too [a nationwide support group] meeting, they asked if anyone at the meeting had a prosthesis. When Tom said he did, a doctor who had prostate cancer came over to talk with him about it, and he told him what could be done to make it better. After the meeting, Tom came home all excited about the new techniques, and the very next night we made love. It made all the difference in the world.

The three main options for artificially inducing an erection—vacuum pump, drug injection, and penile implant (prosthesis)—are described separately on the following pages. Each of them has been widely used by posttreatment prostate cancer patients, most of whom, when surveyed, have reported a high degree of satisfaction. There are numerous variations of each option, so be sure to explore all possibilities thoroughly with your doctor

◊ *vacuum pump:* The easiest nonsurgical means of artificially producing a strong erection is by using a vacuum pump. Essentially, a vacuum pump consists of a rigid tubelike structure that is slid over the penis and barricaded in such a manner that the air inside is sealed off. Then, a pumplike mechanism is used to create a partial vacuum inside the tube, thus forcing blood to flow into the penis and fully engorge it. Usually the pumping process takes from one to two minutes, but it may take longer.

This kind of device comes in many different forms and is known by many different names, including "constrictor," "tensor," and "suction cyl-inder." Most models feature a ring that fits snugly around the base of the penis and helps to create the air seal during the pumping process. The ring then remains on the penis after the tube is removed to help keep blood from flowing back out of the engorged penis tissue. The ring can usually be worn without discomfort or unpleasant side effects for up to thirty minutes at a time. Some models of this device feature hand pumps (a squeezable bulb), while others have battery-driven pumps.

It takes a while for a man to feel comfortable and proficient using a vacuum pump—anytime from a few days of regular use to a few weeks. There is certainly some loss of spontaneity in begin-ning a sexual interlude with a couple minutes of pumping; but, to the ultimate delight of many men and their partners, the quality of the erection is very good, and the penetration itself feels completely natural. A few men, after having used the vacuum pump for an extended period, have even reported experiencing occasional natural erections for the first time since treatment. However, medical science considers the likelihood of a patient's having this type of response to be very slim. It is definitely *not* a reasonable expectation.

In some cases, men who use vacuum pumps do experience minor, temporary side effects that necessitate two or three days of nonuse followed by more careful use. These include:

1. the appearance of tiny reddish dots on the sur-face of the penis, sometimes accompanied by a mildly unpleasant hypersensitivity (a condition known as "petechiae," caused by too rapidly engorging the penis);

2. temporary bruising anywhere on the penis, but especially at the base (a condition known as

"ecchymosis," caused by keeping the penis under vacuum pressure for too long).

Although the vacuum pump is generally quite safe, there are some circumstances in which it *may* have to be used with extra caution: for example, if the user has blood-clotting problems or sickle-cell anemia. Whatever the circumstances, any potential user should first consult with his doctor just to make sure it's okay.

◊ *injection:* Another, less common approach to inducing an erection artificially involves the patient injecting himself at the base of the penis with one of three different types of medications: *papaverine*, a drug that doctors often use to create an erection for diagnostic purposes; *phentolamine*, an alpha-blocker; or *prostaglandin El*, a muscle relaxant that has the effect of drawing blood into the penis. The injection process itself is easy and relatively painless, yielding (usually) a high-quality erection within a few minutes that can last an hour or even more.

   Unfortunately, there are also major drawbacks associated with penile injections. In most cases, the drugs can safely be used only at certain intervals of time: anywhere from once a day to once every three or four days. If they're used improperly, they can sometimes produce a long-lasting and uncomfortable erection (a condition known as "priapism") that may even require medical attention. And, in rare circumstances, serious side effects may occur, such as elevated blood pressure, heart palpitations, liver complications, and fibrosis (the buildup of scar tissue at the site of injection).

   Patients who choose to self-administer penile injections must place themselves under the supervision of their doctor in order to obtain the drug(s) they are using. Often, a doctor will recommend regular, periodic testing for such a patient to help guarantee that no injection related problems are occurring and that the drug dosage remains appropriate. Doctors also occasionally recommend that a patient use a combination of vacuum pump and injection to achieve an erection, so that the drug dosage can be reduced and the risk of negative side effects minimized.

◊ *penile implants:* The third approach to inducing an erection artificially involves having a mechanical device (or "prosthesis") surgically implanted in the man's penis, by means of which he can create an erection on demand. It's clearly the most radical approach—it's invasive and permanently changes the interior of the penis—but in many respects it can also be the most satisfactory, depending on the situation. There are three basic types of penile implants:

1. *the semirigid implant*

   This is the simplest type of implant: A silicone-coated metal or fiber rod (sometimes a pair of rods) is implanted inside the penis so that it is always erect. When the man is not engaged in sexual intercourse, the rod can be bent—by bending the penis itself—so that the penis hangs downward (although there may still be a noticeable bulge that needs to be concealed by loose clothing or special underwear).

   A major advantage of this type of implant is that it is relatively easy to install (often the operation can be performed on an outpatient basis), and there are rarely any complications. Typically, the user can engage in satisfactory penetration within four to six weeks after implantation. The only significant disadvantage—besides, possibly, an ever-present bulge—is the fact that the artificial erection involves no blood engorgement, which means that the penis does not increase in length or girth from its flaccid state, and as a result, the sensation of having an erection for the man is not quite the same (although still very pleasant).

A recently developed, more sophisticated version of the semirigid implant features a spring-loaded metal cable running through an interlocking series of plastic blocks. When the cable is bent into the downward flaccid position, the spring is disengaged and the cable hangs limp. Thus, the penis doesn't bulge at all but looks perfectly natural. When the cable is bent upward, the spring is activated, causing the cable to lock. Regrettably, the increase in sophistication also means an increase in the possibility of complications, such as mechanical breakdowns or infections.

2. *The self-contained inflatable implant*
As opposed to the semirigid implant described above, the self-contained inflatable implant is a more complex single-unit mechanism consisting of two sealed, inflatable cylinders containing fluid (positioned down the length of the penis) and a twin-pump mechanism (located beneath the head—or glans—of the penis). When the man wants to induce an erection, he squeezes the head of his penis, and the pumps move fluid from a storage section of each cylinder into the main compartment. When he wants to lose the erection, he bends his penis near the glans, and the fluid runs back into the storage section of each cylinder.

The advantages of a self-contained inflatable implant are impressive. The penis looks and feels natural in its flaccid, erecting, and erect states (although it does not increase in length or girth when erect). What's even more attractive to many users is that this kind of implant provides the outward illusion of having an almost natural erecting experience—with no visible mechanical aids. A man's partner can even enjoy "stimulating" the erection herself.

The disadvantages of the self-contained inflatable implant result from its complexity. The implantation surgery usually requires a one- to two-day stay in the hospital, followed by approximately six weeks of healing before the implant can actually be used. Compared to other implants, it's more difficult for the patient to operate. The implant can also fail: Approximately five percent of users need to return for another, restorative operation within the first five years. Finally, there is the rare but serious possibility of infection due to fluid leakage from the implant cylinders.

3. *The fully (or "multicomponent") inflatable implant*
The fully inflatable implant, like the self-contained inflatable implant described above, consists mainly of two inflatable cylinders and a pumping mechanism. However, in the fully inflatable device, the storage cylinders are "balloon-style" ones that give the erect penis extra girth and (with some models) extra length, as in a natural erection, although no actual blood engorgement is involved.

Another way that the fully inflatable device differs from the self-contained one is that the fluid reservoir in the fully inflatable device is usually located in the lower abdomen, and the pump, in the scrotum: with flexible tubing connecting them together, as well as linking the pump to the two cylinders. When an erection is desired, the man (or his partner) squeezes the "inflation" section of the scrotum pump for about thirty seconds. To lose the erection, he (or she) squeezes the "deflation" section of the pump for a similar amount of time.

The fully inflatable implant is the most natural feeling and performing of all the implants, but it is also the most complicated. The hospital stay and recuperation time are about the same as for the self-contained device (although the surgery itself is more involved), but the fully inflatable device has a slightly higher failure rate—mainly because there are more places where leakage can potentially occur.

"Manhood" Issues

Many men come through the experience of prostate cancer treatment with their overall sense of manhood intact. For some, it's even enhanced. They have just made it through a life-or-death crisis that challenged their courage, endurance, and stamina: an acid test of manhood. A few men may even say to themselves with pride, as actor and cancer patient John Wayne, a macho icon, once did: "I've licked the big C!"

However, many men do *not* feel as secure about their manhood after prostate cancer treatment as they did before. This is especially true if they are newly faced with temporary, chronic, or permanent impotence. It isn't simply a question of a man having too much of his identify wrapped up in his penis. For a man *or* a woman, sex is so involved with gender that the two terms are hopelessly confused in most languages (in English, for example, even formal application forms ask, colloquially, what "sex" the applicant is, when, technically, the accurate term is "gender"). Thus, a man who loses sexual desire and even a certain amount of sexual function is likely to experience a simultaneous loss of identity and, as a possible consequence, feel baffled, helpless, embarrassed, humiliated, ashamed, and even guilty.

Closely tied to sex are other issues associated with "manhood" that also become problematic after prostate cancer treatment. One of these issues is *control*. Typically—one might even say stereotypically—a man is expected to maintain control over his life, just as he is expected to maintain control over the sex act (and, for that matter, over "*his* woman"). His recent bout with cancer followed by his altered life after—or during—treatment throws into question his ability to maintain any kind of control at all.

Then there's the issue of intimacy. A man is socially conditioned to be—or at least to appear to be—strong, silent, and unemotional: a person of action, not words and feelings. For many men, sex is their primary mode of communicating intimately with their mate. For some men, regrettably, it's their only mode. Whatever the case, when sex becomes difficult for a man, so does his ability to be close to his mate in what he considers to be a "masculine" way.

To make matters worse, the man has been living through a period of serious illness that has probably forced him to be much less private and self-reliant than he likes to be. Now that things have stabilized somewhat, he may want to avoid as much "unnecessary" intimacy as he can with his partner. His conscious or subconscious mind may feel that this is the only way he can get over his embarrassing state of dependence and recapture his former, more macho sense of self. Alternatively, because he doesn't have many nonsexual intimacy skills at his disposal, he may allow himself to drift along in a state of childlike dependence on his partner, unable for the time being to figure out how to establish a more adult, masculine relationship with her.

The way to help your partner cope with any of these difficulties relating to his sense of "manhood" is to exercise compassionate understanding and to do what you can, tactfully, to express your love and regard whenever the opportunity arises. Perhaps the single best strategy you can employ is to encourage him to talk with you more often: not only about his posttreatment coping problems, but also about anything else. It's an excellent means of rebuilding or strengthening the intimate bonds between you. Your partner may feel self-conscious if you repeatedly refer to how manly you think he is, but a few well-timed indications are definitely in order.

You might also try slowly but surely incorporating more romance into your lives: hand-in-hand walks at sunset, impromptu picnics in the park, festive nights out on the town, weekends at a nearby inn. Buy one of the many "relationship" books now on the market for some suggestions, and don't forget to try some of the "Beyond the Erection" activities listed earlier in this chapter. Take heart from these two testimonials offered by a caregiver and a patient (not a couple) who were interviewed for this book:

> In many ways, our life together after the cancer has changed for the better. We value each other more, and so we've opened up more. We talk more, we touch more, we spend more time together. There's a welcome mellowness that wasn't there before.
>
> —a fifty-eight-year-old wife of a patient

> When I first found out I was impotent and going to stay that way, I didn't feel one iota of sexual interest. I hated even thinking about sex. But that passed. My wife and I found new ways of doing things. Now, I think about sex more than I did before, and I enjoy that. Actually, I never really thought about sex before, I just did it. What a waste!
>
> —a sixty-four-year-old patient

A final, but supremely important, piece of advice is to care for yourself just as well as you care for your partner. At all times in a relationship, but particularly during sex-related crises like the ones we've been examining, women need to guard against losing their own sense of self and "womanhood" by overidentifying with their mate's difficulties.

Much too often (due in large part to their own social conditioning) women tend to blame themselves for their partner's low self-esteem or poor sexual appetite. They feel that it must have something to do with their lack of "feminine" appeal. They accuse themselves of being too passive and unprovocative one moment, and too assertive and threatening another moment. In reality, the source of the problem lies in the man's own sense of self—independent of his mate or his relationship, however much either may fall short of perfection or wind up being hurt.

As a caregiver for a man concerned about his masculinity and perhaps incapable of performing sexually in a manner that's mutually satisfying, you will have your own set of worries and frustrations. If at all possible and appropriate, you should try to share your personal concerns with your partner. After all, you're asking him to share his troubles with you, and it just may inspire him to offer you some masculine comfort! Dr. William Masters, the pioneer authority on sex, describes two-way conversation about such matters as the most rewarding type of communication that an intimate relationship can offer: "It's the privilege of exchanging vulnerabilities."

If this kind of sharing seems inappropriate or undesirable to you, given the present situation, then be sure to discuss your problems with a close, trusted friend, your doctor, or a professional counselor before they get even worse. The more secure, confident, and competent you feel, the better able you will be to help instill security, confidence, and competence in your partner.

Sensuality

Any serious physical illness can shatter a person's trust in his or her body and therefore diminish his or her capacity to enjoy that body. Cancer—still so strongly associated in our culture with dread, horror, uncleanness, and even (irrationally) contagion—can have an especially devastating impact on a person's "body sense". There may come a time in a cancer patient's life when all known cancerous tissue has been cut, blasted, or burned out of the body, but there's *always* the possibility of recurrence. Thus, in the cancer patient's mind, the body somehow still remains a battlefield rather than a playground.

A man who has just undergone treatment for prostate cancer is understandably going to be preoccupied with his capacity to give and receive *sexual* pleasure. But a person's sensuality involves much more than what we narrowly define as "sexuality." It includes all the ways that we can derive joy and satisfaction from our senses: seeing, hearing, smelling, tasting, and touching, as well as dancing, singing, smiling, adventuring, and even resting. It's the manner in which we feel, express, and cultivate our sense of aliveness.

To help rekindle your mate's sensuality (and, in the process, enhance his sexuality), slowly but surely guide him toward experiences that are rich in sensory stimulation—anything from simple exercises that get the body moving, to playful water-pistol fights, to extravagantly indulgent nights of feasting or afternoons at a spa. Review the following features in this book for some ideas to get your started: "Dr. Barbara and Dr. Sandy's TakeCare Tips" (chapter 8), "Healthy Exercise" (chapter 8), and "Beyond the Erection" (chapter 9).

Continence

(For more specific information about the risks of incontinence related to specific treatments, see chapters 6 and 8.)

Despite the value that men in general place on being able to have an erection, clinical and anecdotal evidence increasingly indicates that posttreatment prostate cancer patients are far more worried about their ability to control urination. A two-year study of such patients released in 1993 by Dr. Mark Litwin, a professor of urology and public health at the University of California at Los Angeles, supports this conclusion. Referring to his study, Litwin remarked:

> Being able to control urination is a "quality of life" issue that has far more significance than is commonly acknowledged for all adults, but especially for men over fifty: men who are within the prostate-cancer age range.

A prostate cancer patient's incontinence can mean much more to him than the day-after-day, all-day and all-night threat of inconvenience, embarrassment, and discomfort related to urination. It can also serve as a very tangible reminder that he no longer has the control over his life that he once had. Furthermore, it can keep fueling his fear of cancer and his despair that he will never be able to trust his body—or his coping capacities—again.

But the picture isn't always so bleak. Many posttreatment prostate cancer patients rise to the quirky challenges of incontinence with great fortitude, pluck, and even humor. One of these men is the singer-actor Robert Goulet. Diagnosed with prostate cancer in 1993, he immediately had a prostatectomy; three weeks later, to the amazement of everyone, he was playing King Arthur in a revival tour of the Lerner and Loewe musical *Camelot*, even though he was suffering postoperative pain and total incontinence. In a February 1994 appearance on ABC-TV's *Good Morning America* program, he recalled an incident during this tour:

> Unfortunately, for most of the show I had to wear tights. Of course, given the situation, they were very dark, very heavily padded tights! Well, right in the middle of the show, there's a scene where I'm all alone on center stage, standing on top of a small hill, spotlit, with my legs spread, singing my heart out. I hit one particular high note, and, sure enough, my bladder gushed away. I could feel my eyes widening. I didn't think the audience could actually tell what had happened, but after the show, I asked Patricia Keyes, my costar, if she noticed anything, well, strange, during that song. And she said, "There was nothing obvious, Robert, but when I saw that twinkle in your eye, I knew it meant a tinkle down your thigh."

Men who are best able to deal with their incontinence are men who can put the situation into proportion: yes, it may be a big *problem*, but how much of a *bother* is that problem? For instance, a man may have the big problem of not being able to control his urination at all—the same problem Robert Goulet had; but with the help of comfortable absorbent pads (described later in this chapter), this problem may rarely actually bother him.

It's easy in this type of situation for a man to get more upset than he needs to be. After all, the whole idea of not having urinary control is in itself difficult for him to accept, and the sensation of involuntarily voiding urine is a very strange one. But with a little "attitude adjustment," he can learn to take things as they come without getting unduly discouraged or panic stricken. On the following pages, "Problem versus Bother" offers an exercise that may help your partner in this endeavor.

It's also easy for the caregiver to experience unnecessary anxiety relating to her partner's incontinence. Try not to feel too worried if you find yourself plagued by doubts and fears regarding your future as a couple or even your husband's masculinity. It's only natural that these feelings should emerge, given the way that the human mind reacts to anything unusual.

A forty-year-old spouse interviewed for this book remembered having a nightmare that made her realize just how much her image of her husband's masculinity was being subconsciously affected by his incontinence:

> I woke up with this awful picture of a man with no sexual organ. Instead, he had a diaper that became continuous with his skin. That dream left a profound impression! I just hadn't been facing how much it disturbed me to see my husband wearing sweatpants during the day and a nightshirt at night. When he started wearing regular pants, I felt so much better. I caught myself thinking, *Oh, he's come back! That's great.*

When you notice that you're having similar mental images or thoughts, acknowledge them for what they are—inevitable responses during a time of change and uncertainty. Above all, try to guard against feeling guilty or ashamed. You have a right to your private thoughts, and these kinds of thoughts are perfectly understandable. Just be careful not to confuse the things that you imagine with the things that are actually true.

Bear in mind that this kind of exercise can also be applied to issues relating to impotence.

As for the man himself, aside from adjusting his attitude, what can he do to cope with incontinence as effectively as possible? More to the point, how can he best work toward overcoming it?

First of all, it helps to understand exactly what is going on: the manner in which the urinary system *normally* functions, and why it isn't functioning that way now. The urinary system consists of the kidneys, ureters, bladder, and urethra. The kidneys, filtering the bloodstream for impurities, manufacture urine as a waste product and then release it into the bladder through the

Problem versus Bother

As part of his 1993 study of incontinent prostate cancer patients, UCLA's Dr. Mark Litwin asked his subjects to distinguish between how big each specific continence-related *problem* was, and how much *bother* that problem actually caused. For example, in regard to urinary leakage (a common continencerelated problem), a man might say that his frequency rate was very high (a "major" problem), but he wasn't actually troubled by it very much because of the pads he wore (a "minor" bother). Litwin's purpose was to enable such men to differentiate between the severity oftheir situation in itself, and the actual quality of life they were experiencing while in that situation. Here are some questions that can get your partner to start making this type of important, quality-of-life distinction:

(The user rates his response to each question in the blank space that follows: 1=minor, up to 4=major.)

1. *Problem:* How often do you leak urine?: (1) never or rarely; (2) weekly; (3) once a day; (4) more than once a day _____
   Bother: How often does this cause you significant physical discomfort or embarrassment?: (1) never or rarely; (2) occasionally; (3) frequently; (4) every time

   _____

2. *Problem:* How often do you have to put on some kind of absorbent product?: (1) once a week (2) several days each week; (3) once a day; (4) twice a day or more _____
   Bother: How much trouble does this procedure usually cause you?: (1) none; (2) very little; (3) a considerable amount; (4) a great deal _____

3. *Problem:* How many activities are you incapable of performing because of your incontinence?: (1) none; (2) a few; (3) a significant number; (4) a very large number

   _____

Bother: How much are you usually upset or inconvenienced by this incapability?: (1) not at all; (2) a little; (3) a considerable amount; (4) a great deal _____

4. *Problem:* How often do you leak urine during sex?: (1) never; (2) rarely; (3) occasionally; (4) frequently

_____

Bother: How much shame, embarrassment, or trouble does this usually cause you?: (1) none; (2) a little; (3) a fair amount; (4) a great deal _____

ureters. It's an ongoing process that accelerates whenever we drink liquids or otherwise consume fluids. The average daily production of urine totals about a half gallon. The bladder can expand to absorb about one and a half to three cups of urine at a time (depending on the individual) before it sends a signal to the brain that the stored urine needs to be released. Normally, despite this signal, the bladder will continue to receive and store urine without registering too much discomfort until it's convenient for the person to urinate.

In a man's body, two voluntarily controlled urinary sphincters are responsible for this retention:

1. the *internal sphincter*, located at the base of the bladder right before the prostate gland; and

2. the *external sphincter*, located at the opposite end of the prostate gland, where it forms part of the so-called "pelvic floor" muscles that, among other functions, serve as a sling to keep the bladder lifted.

When it's convenient for a man to urinate, both sphincters are voluntarily relaxed, along with the pelvic floor muscles, and the bladder-stored urine runs into the urethra, which transports the urine down through the penis and out of the body. (For drawings that depict many of these anatomical features, see chapter 2.)

When a man's prostate gland is surgically removed—the treatment for prostate cancer that most frequently results in incontinence—so is the internal sphincter. This leaves only the external sphincter, in cooperation with the other pelvic floor muscles, to hold back urine in the bladder.

So, what can the postprostatectomy man, or any man suffering incontinence, do to cope with his condition and, hopefully, regain more control over his urinary function? He should be sure to consult with his doctor at frequent and regular intervals, especially if he is taking any medication (which might adversely affect his condition) or if he is overweight (which creates more strain on the bladder). He should also consider getting a second opinion. Here are some other guidelines:

⬥ He should try to drink at least two quarts of fluids (a high percentage of which should be water) per day—a normal healthy intake. Many people suffering from incontinence falsely assume that minimizing their fluid consumption will help alleviate their incontinence problem. In reality, it may worsen it: causing dark, thick urine that is more uncomfortable to hold and to pass, and perhaps triggering constipation.

It *is* a good idea for him to limit or avoid fluid consumption in the evening, so that he'll be less likely to be bothered by the need to urinate during the night. For the same basic reason, it's also wise for him to limit or avoid fluid consumption an hour before, and during, important outings, meetings, or tasks during the day.

Above all, he should avoid consuming more fluids than he needs (i.e., beyond the two-quart recommendation), and he should put especially strict limits on his intake of alcohol, caffeinated coffee, and caffeinated soft drinks, which compel a person to want to urinate more frequently. Grapefruit and grapefruit juice also have this effect.

⬥ He should perform "Kegel exercises" to strengthen his pelvic floor muscles. Named for Dr. Arnold H.

Kegel, an American gynecologist who developed them to help women overcome incontinence after giving birth, these exercises work on that particular muscle group that a continent person consciously strains in order to start or stop the urine flow. The "strain" sensation itself is, for the man, a slight constriction felt somewhere in the area between the anus and the scrotum.

There are two types of Kegel exercises: "quick" Kegels and "slow" Kegels. Each consists of first tightening and then relaxing these muscles (without simultaneously contracting the abdomen or rectum). Quick Kegels are done rapidly, slow Kegels involve holding the contraction while counting to four.

A typical exercise regimen might include four repetitions of each type of Kegel exercise every couple of hours. However, a Patient's specific regimen can be whatever he wants it to be, as long as he performs it fairly frequently and sticks to it, day after day. Because a person can perform a Kegel while sitting or standing without an observer being able to tell, many men simply do an isolated Kegel every now and then when they think about it. Others make a point of doing at least a couple of Kegels every hour.

Whatever regimen your partner chooses, he should try performing several Kegels at least one or two times each day *while* he is urinating: i.e., he should actually try to stop and start the urine flow several times. The more the exercise is practiced, the more aware of that particular muscle group he will become, and the stronger that muscle group can get. Like any muscle-building exercise, it requires faith and perseverance: it may take two or three months before the results are noticeable.

Other options for regaining control over bladder function involve artificial procedures or devices that may or, may not be appropriate for a particular situation. They include:

◊ *collagen implants:* A collagen implant is, simply put, an injection of highly purified collagen (from animal tissue) into the tissues surrounding the urethra. This adds bulk to the urethra, so that it can close more tightly and thus help prevent involuntary urine leakage. One of the most common brands of collagen implants is called "Contigen," which features connective tissue from cow bones.

A patient relying on collagen implants will need to be reinjected periodically: anywhere from one to seven treatments for the first year, followed by less frequent treatments in subsequent years, varying according to the individual patient and the success of the procedure. In a small percentage of cases, there may be allergic or infectious complications, but generally it's quite safe. Usually it is not advised (because it may be useless) if the patient has been bothered by sustained or occasional incontinence for less than twelve months, or if his incontinence-related problems have shown any significant improvement during the last twelve months.

◊ *artificial sphincter implants:* A doughnut-shaped hydraulic prosthesis is surgically implanted around the urethra to replace the now missing internal sphincter (formerly between the bladder and the prostate gland). It is attached by thin tubing to a bulb implanted in the scrotum. When the man wants to urinate, he squeezes his scrotum where the bulb lies, and this action drains fluid from the artificial sphincter so that it opens, releasing urine from the bladder. Several minutes after the bladder has emptied, the sphincter automatically refills and closes off the bladder.

The implantation procedure usually requires a two- to three-day hospital stay, and there is a 20 percent risk of complications during the first year after installation, most of them involving minor infections or discomfort. However, the implant has a high rate of success (90 percent). Furthermore, it is often possible for a man to have both a penile implant and an artificial sphincter implant without any resulting problems or any visible evidence of either device.

◊ *collection systems:* The purpose of a collection system is not exactly to help a man *control* urination, but, rather, to help him experience *uncontrolled* urination in a more pleasant, less messy or embarrassing manner. Most systems feature a rubber shaft (connected to a waistbelt) that is bound to the penis so that it can funnel urine through a drainage tube into a collection bag secured to one of the man's legs.

Users must be careful to attach the penis shaft in such a way that it doesn't either fall off inadvertently or constrict circulation in the penis. They must also make special efforts to keep themselves— and the apparatus— clean, so that there's no risk of infection.

◊ *electrostimulation sessions or implants:* In some cases, the administration of small, relatively painless electrical shocks to the exterior sphincter has proved helpful in building up the sphincter muscles. These shocks can be administered during regular office visits to a physician or via a battery-powered implant. Electrostimulation for this purpose is still in the pioneer stage of development, so not much is presently known about its long-range capabilities or side effects.

◊ *experimental procedures:* Among the possible procedures to remedy incontinence that are still being researched and developed are: reconstructive surgery, drug injections, and biofeedback monitoring. Ask your doctor if any of these procedures might be appropriate for the patient's situation.

It is encouraging to remember that the majority of patients who experience incontinence immediately after a prostatectomy (or, for that matter, after *any* form of prostate cancer treatment) are able to recover a satisfactory level of continence within a year. Many recover without doing anything special to assist the recovery; others recover only after conscientiously performing muscle-building exercises for an extended period of time. Some can achieve one hundred percent recovery of their former continence, and a few even manage to build up more urinary control than they had before the illness struck!

To be sure, regaining continence is often a slow, gradual process. During this time, besides (possibly) needing to use underpads and drawsheets on the bed, the patient will have to wear some sort of absorbent product(s) to take care of urinary leaks.

Ask your doctor for advice about particular absorbent product(s) to use, and then experiment. Typically, a patient will use several different types of products over the same time period, since one type may be more appropriate for a certain activity or occasion than another. He will also progress from relying primarily on highly absorbent products to using increasingly less absorbent (and thus less bulky) products as he regains more and more control over his urination. The different generic types of products are described below; various commercial brands—such as Secure, Depend, Attends, and Dignity—may offer additional, specialized types:

- ◊ *pads:* Also called "guards" or "shields," these are padded strips (sometimes with gel inserts) that are worn inside brief-style underwear, between the legs and over the penis. They provide the most mobility with the least visibility, so many men use them, for example, when they're out in public wearing thin or relatively tightfitting clothing.

- ◊ *pad-and-pant systems:* These systems contain coordinating pads and brief-style pants. The pads are tucked into the pants, which are worn in place of— or underneath—conventional underwear. Like pads alone, they provide maximum mobility with minimum visibility.

◊ *absorbent ("fitted") briefs:* A prefitted, brief-style pant is itself absorbent, with no need for a separate pad. It's much more absorbent than a pad-and-pant system, but it's also significantly bulkier, so it's usually not worn in public except under loose-fitting clothes.

◊ *absorbent pants or undergarments:* Of all absorbent products of this nature, undergarments, which are bound in place by the user, are the most effective and the bulkiest. They are typically only worn at home or while sleeping, for maximum protection.

◊ *children's diapers:* Some men prefer to use large-size disposable children's diapers rather than any of the above-described products because they are more absorbent. They also tend to be less expensive. However, they are bulkier and more awkward to wear as well.

Peace of Mind

Prostate cancer patients and their caregivers naturally look forward to the end of treatment as a time when they can finally relax and resume some sort of "normal" life again. In fact, many of them are surprised to discover that their anxiety levels *rise* instead of fall after the treatment is over.

During the time that the treatment is in progress, the patient and his caregiver have a definite sense of "doing something" about the cancer. They are surrounded and actively supported by a medical team, relatives, and friends; and they can temporarily justify putting all other cares and concerns on hold. Then, after treatment, they're pretty much on their own again. A crisis may have passed, but it's left new worries and new problems in its wake. Meanwhile, all the other cares and concerns that they disregarded during the crisis come back crying for attention.

Dr. Jimmie Holland, a leading psychiatrist at the Memorial Sloan-Kettering Cancer Center in New York City—an institution that offers the country's largest training program in psychiatric oncology—spoke of this type of emotional "downtrend" for the patient in an interview published by *The New York Times* on July 20, 1993 ("Listening to the Emotional Needs of Cancer Patients," by Elisabeth Rosenthal):

> Most people think of themselves as invulnerable, but people who have had cancer cannot think like that. Many feel . . . like a sword of Damocles is hanging over their heads. They have a sense that they're damaged goods. You'd expect people to feel good when they finish treatment, but from their perspective, the medicine [or surgery] that has kept the disease at bay has stopped and they are not going to see their doctor, who has been their ally in fighting the disease every week.

To make matters worse, situations that weren't previously acknowledged as problems by the patient and/or his caregiver may now seem very troublesome indeed. A loathsome job that the patient was simply performing for the sake of retirement benefits may suddenly seem unendurable. A caregiver may no longer be capable of suppressing her dissatisfaction with the community in which they live. A waning sex life that was tolerated in silence by both partners before the illness may, afterward, become an unavoidable topic of their daily conversation. And their fear of aging—formerly confined to the back of their minds—may now start staring them right in the face.

In many respects, the posttreatment period can feature the same kinds of adverse emotional reactions as the pretreatment period did, including anger, fear, depression, mourning, guilt, resentment, and entitlement. For this reason, it may be helpful to review the coping strategies for patients and caregivers that are offered in chapter 5, "Dealing with the Diagnosis: Emotional Issues," especially keeping a journal and breathing for relaxation.

Sometimes, what is commonly called depression—recurring feelings of sadness and despair—can develop into what is clinically called depression: a much more serious and multifaceted condition that is in fact a distinct psychiatric disorder. Fortunately, clinical depression can be successfully treated with medication and/or psychotherapy, and early diagnosis greatly increases the odds of a complete recovery.

If your partner or you experience four or more of the following twelve symptoms of clinical depression for over three weeks, you should consult with a doctor, psychiatrist, psychologist, or mental health specialist:

Twelve Symptoms of Clinical Depression

1. a persistent sad, anxious, or "empty" mood

2. a loss of interest or pleasure in activities that, up until recently, you enjoyed

3. an ongoing fatigue or decrease in physical energy

4. sleep-related problems, like insomnia, oversleeping, or early awakening

5. eating-related problems, like loss of appetite, recurrent cravings, weight loss, or weight gain

6. mind-related difficulties, like not being able to concentrate, remember things, or make decisions

7. excessive crying

8. recurring aches and pains that are otherwise inexplicable and that don't respond to treatment

9. lingering or recurring feelings of hopelessness or pessimism

10. lingering or recurring feelings of guilt, worthlessness, or helplessness

11. ongoing irritability

12. thoughts, talk, or actions indicating suicidal feelings

The last symptom—thoughts, talk, or actions indicating suicidal feelings—is especially serious all by itself. Never ignore or underestimate it. Instead, seek advice from a doctor, psychiatrist, psychologist, or mental health professional as soon as possible.

Here are some other guidelines that you and your partner can follow to maintain peace of mind during the potentially very difficult first year after treatment:

◊ *Recognize and accept that certain things are going to be different for both of you—individually and as a couple— than they were before the illness.* It's unrealistic to expect that you can simply pick up where you left off before the illness. Too much has happened, externally and internally.

  As a caregiver, you need to be particularly careful to avoid becoming determined and devoted to getting back the man you knew before. Your well-meaning efforts could actually stymie his recovery: deep down, he may know all too well that he's simply not, and can never be, the same man he used to be. But that doesn't mean he can't become a well-adjusted, self-confident "new" man, able to enjoy himself, his life, and his partner—and able to be enjoyed, in turn, by you.

◊ *Seek pleasure, control, and intimacy when and where you can.* The more you actively look for ways to experience pleasure, a sense of control over your fate, and emotional intimacy with your partner and other important people in your life, the more certain you are to find them. Be patient and perseverant (respecting your personal limits!). You may learn, much to your initial dismay, that the old ways by which you went about obtaining these qualities in your life are no longer possible, which means that you'll have to find new ways.

  For example, your partner's weakened or compromised physical condition may preclude skiing, a former source of pleasure, so you could try long walks in the snow instead. Due to the way that cancer has disrupted your life, you and your partner

individually may no longer feel that you have the
same control over your future that you had before;
however, exercising more control over your day-to-
day health could help make up for that loss. And,
because of treatment-related sexual complications,
you and your partner as a couple may not be able to
generate the exact same sensations of physical intimacy that you did before; but you could certainly
become just as emotionally intimate—or more so—
by trying out other ways of being physically close.

◊ *Cultivate positive thoughts and behaviors, but don't feel
that you have to be positive all the time.* There's no
denying that it helps to be as upbeat, optimistic, and
easygoing as you reasonably can. However, each
person has a limit for enforced positivism that he or
she should respect and not be ashamed to admit.

During the same interview quoted above, Dr.
Holland of the Memorial Sloan-Kettering Cancer
Center had this to say about the popular notion that
cancer patients *must* think positively in order to deal
with their illness or their life after illness:

> Patients get bombarded by family members
> who say, "You aren't trying hard enough." I
> think we're overdoing it, trying to make every-
> one into a Ihappy warrior. Some people are not
> good at it. Each of us has a different style of
> coping, and many work equally well.

◊ *Explore psychological and spiritual resources that can
help you lead a more satisfying life.* If, during the
course of the illness, you haven't already established
an ongoing relationship with a psychotherapist or a
spiritual counselor, now is an ideal time to do so,
when you and your partner are struggling to lay the
foundations for a new phase in your life as individuals and as a couple. Even on your own, there
are books you can read and classes you can take
that can offer you invaluable assistance in regaining

your emotional equilibrium. Ask around and get some suggestions.

A sixty-five-year-old patient interviewed for this book shared this inspiring story about a coping technique he learned from an adult education workshop given by a local college:

> I would always shy away from anything that seemed "New Age," but then my wife signed the two of us up for a weekend retreat called "Personal Empowerment." Well, we were taught many different things, some of which I could take or leave, but there was this one thing that stayed with me and that really seems to work. I just close my eyes, and picture a flame coming out of a small hole in the ground, an eternal flame. This is my will to live. And I just watch it, knowing it won't go out. I let this image mesmerize me. And you know what? It never fails to make me feel calmer and more confident.

10

Back to Your Future

- ◊ Renewing your postcrisis life

- ◊ Starting or joining a support group

- ◊ Advocating for research, detection, and treatment

- ◊ Resources for patients and their partners

Life after prostate cancer—for the patient, for the caregiver, and for the patient-caregiver couple—can be better than it was before, or it can be an unending nightmare of mourning the past, hating the present, and fearing the future. The way to make it better rather than worse is to keep focusing, as much as possible, on what *heals*, instead of brooding on what *hurts*.

At least for a while, the cancer crisis is behind you and your partner. You've had a chance to mourn the loss of your pre-illness lifestyle and to appreciate how precious life really is. Now is the time to take control over your destiny once again. It doesn't matter how swiftly or gracefully you move, as long as you persevere in moving forward. Otherwise, you'll continue being a victim of the illness by choice rather than necessity.

First, both of you need to tend—gently and lovingly—all of the wounds that the crisis has created: the emotional, spiritual, and interpersonal wounds, as well as the physical ones. This requires ongoing hope, care, understanding, and patience, for the wounds can reopen during any time of stress, illness related or not.

Second, both of you need to cultivate the special insights that the illness ordeal has given you about yourselves and life in general, so that you can make your future years all the richer and more personally fulfilling. In the words of Arthur Keinman, the noted medical sociologist, "Nothing so concentrates experience and clarifies the central conditions of living as serious illness." Having realized this truth for yourselves, you are well equipped to make the most of the life that you have ahead of you—setting good priorities, taking care of the basics, and savoring each moment for what it's worth. It would be a tragic waste simply to throw away your hard-earned wisdom by not acting upon it.

In chapter 1, we examined the difference between *curing* the body and *healing* the person. It's vitally important for you and your partner to stay mindful of that distinction as your lives progress beyond the illness itself. Healing involves actively pursuing a personal sense of "wholeness," so that you come to feel more and more connected to your innermost self and to the life you are leading. It does not mean putting your life on hold, waiting for something to happen that will force the connection. Nor does it mean ignoring your emotions, maintaining an attitude of separateness from the world around you, or functioning according to other people's expectations and beliefs. It means living according to what you feel is best for you.

To sustain the process of healing, you must listen to what your heart and soul have to say, which may require studying their language with new intensity. You must take direction from your own internal sense of things, your intuition, your "gut" feelings. You must seek ways to relate personally to what's going on around you, and let go of ambitions and attitudes that don't suit who you are or the situations in which you find yourself. As you persist in doing these things, your life will gradually bloom with new health.

John Wellwood, a psychotherapist specializing in post-illness recovery, writes in his 1992 book *Ordinary Magie* about the value of looking inward—instead of outward—for guidance in healing:

> It is not surprising that the terms *healing, whole,* and *holy* all come from the same root. When we meet and honor the inner healer—the source of health within us—we initiate a deeper connectedness with ourselves that makes us whole. And this makes us more sensitive to the sacred quality of life—the ordinary magic, beauty, and power at work in our body, our mind, and in all things.

To achieve this kind of inner healing, each of us must work in our own ways, and at our own pace. As a caregiver, you can and should support your partner's healing in a manner that you feel is beneficial for him. You may be able to do him a great deal of good, for example, by encouraging him to express his emotions, to develop positive points of view, and to experiment with life-enhancing activities. But you must be forbearing, tactful, and nonjudgmental in doing so, always respecting his right—and need—to manage his own self-healing process.

Your partner may have to go through a period of silent, perhaps even gloomy, withdrawal before he can muster enough energy to attempt a constructive reengagement with life. Alternatively, he may feel compelled to jump right into a busy schedule, even though you don't think he's ready to do so. Some men thrive on returning to a life that's as near to their precrisis "normal" life as possible. Others find this prospect very intimidating or discouraging, and prefer a life that's different: perhaps more tranquil, perhaps more exciting.

There's no one approach to life after cancer that is right for everyone. If you want to, and if you feel it's appropriate, you should certainly voice your own opinions to your partner about how he might best resume living after the illness crisis. However, you should not feel—or imply in your statements or actions—that your partner needs to follow your advice. He may well be incapable of doing so for reasons that you don't realize and that he can't express. And his own approach may be more effective in the long run than you're capable of recognizing.

In the wake of the illness experience that you and your partner have both endured, the person whom you are most responsible for healing, and most capable of healing, is yourself. Aside from being a caregiver, you are also a person in need of healing that only you can provide. Remember that you, too, have a right to heal in your own way, and at your own pace. Accept and ponder the well-intended, potentially useful advice of your partner, relatives, close friends, health-care professionals, and books like this one, but don't feel that you have to follow such advice if it doesn't seem natural to you.

Every person is unique, and so is every individual case of illness. As the partner of a man who has just fought a battle with a life-threatening cancer that could recur at any time, you are singularly qualified to deal with your situation as you see fit. Doing the best that you can do is, in fact, the best that can be done.

With all of these considerations in mind, you and your partner should each think carefully about how you can utilize the following self-healing recommendations, distilled from the many patient and caregiver interviews conducted for this book:

◊ *Develop and practice regular, private ways to stay in touch with your thoughts and feelings.* The value of keeping a personal, daily journal has already been discussed in this book (see chapter 5). But there are many other ways of monitoring your inner self and drawing from it the inspiration that you need to remain healthy in the fullest sense of the word. Here are some suggestions:

  ◊ Establish a particular place where you go for quiet reflection: both periodically and whenever you feel a special need. It could be a corner of a (relatively) little-used room in your home that you've outfitted with a comfy armchair. Or it could be a park bench, a clearing in a woods, or a quiet spot in a public building that's convenient for quick visits. It should be a place that you reserve—at least primarily—for "thinking things out." If your mind works better when your body's in motion, you can walk a special route that you take for just this purpose (*not* a route that you regularly use for physical exercise). Simply returning to this special place again and again over a period of time will provide a sense of personal stability and give you a better perspective on how your life is going.

◊ Engage in leisure-time activities that foster self-reliance and personal creativity. Ideally, these activities should be strictly for your own private enjoyment, rather than multiperson entertainments (like card games) or lifestyle-related tasks (like cooking). The possibilities include painting, fishing, playing a musical instrument, wood carving, writing poetry, weaving tapestries, learning how to fly.

◊ Ask yourself the following four questions on a regular basis (for example, at the end of each day, on Sunday mornings, or whenever you're feeling down), and answer them as specifically as you can:

1. What have I especially enjoyed [today, this week, recently], and how can I enjoy it more often in the future?

2. What has especially bothered me [today, this week, recently], and what can I do [tomorrow, next week, in the near future] to make it less bothersome?

3. What have I learned [today, this week, recently] that can help me in the future?

4. What can I look forward to [tomorrow, next week, in the near future]?

⬦ *Maintain communication with others.* The single best way to avoid sinking into your own self-made funk is to engage in dialogue with other people—family members, old friends, new friends, and any congenial souls that you encounter during the course of the day. It's also an excellent means of uncovering whole new worlds of information: from what to do about insomnia and where to shop for the freshest produce, to how to laugh at life's little foibles.

Try arranging your schedule so that you regularly get together with people whom you enjoy or with whom you have a lot in common (see, for example, the discussion of support groups under "Resources" later in this chapter). Keep ongoing track of specific things that you'd like to discuss with specific people, as well as general topics for any open-ended conversation. Practice being a good listener whenever you have the chance. Ask your local librarian or bookstore manager to recommend books on enhancing your conversational skills, and periodically review the communication guidelines offered in chapter 5.

⬦ *Generate new life-plans and daily activities based on what the illness experience has taught you.* For many former patients and their caregivers, the illness experience serves as a "wake-up" call—a signal that life doesn't last forever, and that it's time to start doing what they've always wanted to do but have so far put off. If this is your situation, you should begin right away to turn some of your long-cherished dreams into reality. Set several possible goals; make a thorough inventory of your obligations, needs, and resources; and then consult with knowledgeable advisors to determine how best to proceed.

Other patients and caretakers find that their former grand plans for the future are no longer appropriate, due to diminished financial reserves or to new limits on the patients' physical stamina and mobility. If this is your situation, you can still derive a lot of healthy satisfaction from less ambitious, more doable plans. Assuming, for example, that you formerly intended retiring to a life of travel that now seems impractical, you may still be able to set up one or two enjoyable vacations each year. If not, then you should think of other specific pleasures that you can anticipate in the future, such as indulging in a hobby, learning a new skill, or engaging in social activities that you've previously had to deny yourself. The important thing is not just to abandon plans that now seem impossible, but to replace them with new plans.

You may find yourself called upon to make difficult sacrifices especially if you need to take extra care to safeguard your future. A married couple in their mid-sixties who were interviewed for this book felt the need to sell their beloved family home and move into a much smaller co-op apartment that was easier and less expensive to run. They had spent a considerable amount of money because of the husband's prostate cancer, but even more to the point, they had developed concerns about the survivor's ability to manage household affairs should one of them die in the near future. Speaking of this change in living arrangements, and how they were able to accept it philosophically, the wife said:

> Maybe we could have scraped along in our old home, closing off part of it, not keeping the rest of it up as nicely as we had before, and relying on family to help out. But for us, that option was just too depressing. It would have been a day-to-day reminder of how much the illness had reduced our quality of life and our independence. Moving to a new place, even if was smaller and not as nice, became like an

adventure, a new era in our lives. It actually gave us the opportunity to change some of the ways we live for the better. For instance, now we eat our meals in front of a bay window looking out over the treetops, instead of the way we used to, in front of the TV, so there's more talk, more closeness to nature, and more enjoyment of the food.

As this testimony indicates, small changes for the better can go a long way toward rendering life as a whole more worthwhile. Besides making practical adjustments in your major life-plans, you should also try, slowly but surely, to reorganize your day-to-day routines according to what the illness experience has taught you: not only about life values in general, but also about your own specific physical and emotional desires. For example, you may want to include time in each day to exercise, take a nap, phone friends and family, read inspirational books, and/or engage in some form of creative selfexpression, such as writing in a journal, cooking a new kind of meal, or just letting your imagination go as you watch the clouds change shape.

As you move through each day, you may also want to grant yourself a greater degree of personal freedom: the right to sit in the sun and do nothing, to say no to invitations that you don't really want to accept, to dance in the rain for the sheer joy of it, or to complain to your neighbors about their noisy stereo. Let your inner feelings be your guide. When you're tired, rest; when you're full of energy, do something. When you're grateful, give thanks; when you're angry, let it rip.

Any experience of serious illness teaches us that we can't take things for granted. If our goal is to lead a healthier, more wholesome life, we need to live in a more mindful and realistic manner; we can't afford to live in ignorance or self-delusion.

Each and every day, we must accept who we are, appreciate what gives us pain as well as what gives us pleasure, and respect what we cannot do, as well as what we can.

Whether you are a recovering prostate cancer patient or a recovering caregiver, keep in mind that the object of healing is not necessarily to cultivate a *better* self, but, rather, a more *authentic* one. This means honestly admitting, and dealing with, any new weaknesses or needs that you're experiencing.

Marc Ian Barasch, a writer, television producer, and cancer survivor, consulted with hundreds of cancer patients about their life-after-treatment coping strategies for his 1993 best-seller *The Healing Path* (G. P. Putnam's Sons). Repeatedly, his interviewees spoke of the need to embrace—rather than deny, ignore, or fight—the teachings of the illness experience, even though some of those teachings may initially seem negative or even intolerable. What he says below refers specifically to posttreatment patients, but it relates just as well to the partners of such patients:

> Many [patients] said that simply acknowledging the limitations imposed by illness, rather than struggling incessantly against them, felt strangely healing. Carol Boss, an unexpectedly long-term survivor of terminal metastatic breast disease, told me, "We cancer folk are not just shepherds of our strengths, but the custodians of our frailties."

In a subsequent discussion with Barasch, Boss argued that the terms *sickness* and *healing* should be stripped of all language indicating "failure" or "success":

> "It's great to get well," [Boss] said, "but it's not the main thing. All human beings have limited resources. Technically speaking, I'm still in

critical condition; technically, we *all* are. The main thing, I think, is to find a way to live so that your life has real *meaning*."

◊   *Become a healer yourself.* In shamanic cultures, a person who has suffered a serious illness is not considered to be healed until he or she turns into a healer—someone who uses his or her recently acquired knowledge of illness to help others. The effect of this type of process is to transform a negative experience into a positive one, and a passive victim of illness into an active champion of health.

There are many excellent ways for a prostate cancer patient or his companion in suffering to effect this healing transformation in their post-illness lives—doing anything from helping out their own sick family members, friends, and neighbors, to volunteering services at their local hospital, hospice, nursing home, or chapter of the National Cancer Society. But one of the most appropriate things that they can do is to work specifically on behalf of prostate cancer research, detection, and treatment.

That's what Lloyd Ney, a retired engineer in Grand Rapids, Michigan, did a decade ago, after exhaustive radiation and hormone treatments for his prostate cancer that necessitated moving to Canada to receive therapy unavailable in the United States. First, he helped win U.S. federal approval of the Canadian therapy, and then he started PAACT (Patient Advocates for Advanced Cancer Treatment). In 1987, PAACT was incorporated as a ten-thousand-member nonprofit foundation that disseminates treatment-related data to patients and caregivers via a quarterly newsletter and other more comprehensive reports. Ney is particularly concerned about empowering the patient to consider all treatment options, instead of immediately signing up for the most common form of treatment, which is surgery. His mission is distinctly personal and definitely feisty: "The only way we're going to stop the tail from wagging the dog," he asserts, "is to see that the patient is provided with enough information to participate in the decision making."

Another inspiring patient-turned-healer is Edward C. Kaps, a retired industrial relations director for General Motors who, in 1989, suffered a recurrence of his prostate cancer ten years after its initial treatment. In 1990, working closely with his doctor at the University of Chicago Hospital, he invited about three hundred prostate cancer patients to start a support organization. Of the twenty-five men who showed up, five actually formed an ongoing group modeled on the well-known breast cancer support group "Y-Me." Now that small group has evolved into "Us Too," one of the largest and most widespread organizations of its kind, supporting an estimated twenty-five thousand patients and their caregivers in ninety-six chapters across the country.

In 1992, James F. Mullen, a prostate cancer survivor in Sarasota, Florida, started "Man to Man," another nationwide support group, with six men sitting around his dining-room table. That group now has twelve chapters in Florida and sixteen chapters in other states.

And then there's Michael Milken, Wall Street's "junkbond" king in the late 1980s, who discovered he had prostate cancer in 1993 shortly after serving twenty-two months in prison for securities-law violations. No sooner did he start hormone treatment than he began his career as an advocate for prostate cancer research, pledging $5 million toward the creation of Cap Cure (for cancer of the prostate), a foundation that has already sponsored thirty research programs at twenty-five academic medical centers.

If you'd like to launch your own advocacy career—for example, to set up an information exchange, to start a support network, to encourage early detection programs, or to lobby for more research—here are some suggestions:

◊   Begin by talking about your plans with anyone who might be able to supply encouragement, help, or information—including your doctor and the patient representative at your hospital. The more people you bring into the discussion, the more refined and practical your plans will become.

◊   Write a brief statement of your intention to:
The American Self-Help Clearinghouse
St. Clares-Riverside Medical Center
25 Pocono Road
Denville, NJ 07834
This organization can provide you with a "startup" kit and up-to-date lists of state and local clearinghouses for advocacy organizations. Be sure to include a self-addressed, stamped envelope in your letter.

◊   Place an advertisement describing your ambition and asking for help in the "Personals" section of local newspapers and periodicals. Also, investigate computer bulletin board options. CompuServe, the national computer network, runs bulletin boards for people interested in a wide variety of specific illnesses, including prostate cancer. Black Bag, a bulletin board on the FidoNet service, can spread a message to hundreds of local health-related boards throughout the United States. To receive a printout of these boards, send five dollars to:
Edward Del Grosso
29 Golfview Drive, Apt. A-2
Newark, DE 19702

◇ For good step-by-step recommendations on how to set up your own support group, get the booklet "A Guide for Establishing Support Groups," developed by the ICI Pharma Group and the American Foundation for Urologic Disease. It includes sample invitations, press releases, and posters, as well as a list of professional contacts. Consult the ICI Pharma Sales Representative in your area, or call ICI Pharmaceuticals Group, Professional Relations Department, at 1-800-456-3669, extension 7862.

Prostate cancer is a transformational experience for both the patient and the caregiver. Part of this transformation is profoundly disturbing: aside from the physical impact of the illness on the patient, there's the emotional and lifestyle upheaval that affects not just him but everyone around him—especially you. It is our sincere hope that you *and* your partner will use this book, and any other resources you can find, not only to cope with the disturbing part of the transformation but also to realize the potential positive part: a renewal of appreciation for your life, your health, and your relationship.

Resources

Additional Books

Bognar, David. 1998. *Cancer: Increasing Your Odds for Survival*. Berkeley, CA: Hunter House.

Fink, John. 1997. *Third Opinion*. Garden City, New York: Avery Pub Group.

Fugh-Berman, Adriane. 1997. *Alternative Medicine: What Works*. Baltimore: Williams and Wilkins.

Moss, Ralph. 1996. *The Cancer Industry*. Brooklyn, New York: Equinox Press.

———. 1996. *Cancer Therapy*. Brooklyn, New York: Equinox Press.

————. 1997. *Alternative Medicine Online*. Brooklyn, New York: Equinox Press.

Weil, Andrew. 1995. *Natural Health, Natural Medicine*. New York: Houghton Mifflin Company

Medical Search Services

Canhelp (Pat McGrady) 360-437-2291

Healing Choices (Ralph Moss) 718-636-4433

Health Resource 800-949-0900

Schine On-Line Services 800-346-3287

World Wide Web

Cancernet	www.cancernet.nci.nih.gov
Healing Choices (Ralph Moss)	www.ralphmoss.com
Healthfinder	www.healthfinder.com
Herbal Research Foundation	www.herbs.com
Medline	www.nlm.nih.gov
Oncolink	www.oncolink.upenn.edu

Support Groups and Information

The following resources are available to prostate cancer patients and their caregivers at *all* stages of illness and recovery:

Support Groups

Regularly meeting with a support group can be an invaluable source of educational, psychological, and social reinforcement for prostate cancer patients and their caregivers. This remains true even after the illness crisis has passed. Most groups report that up to half their members are people whcse prostate cancer has already been treated and hopefully) removed or arrested.

As forums for giving and getting help, support groups are both highly practical and magically restorative. Mullen, founder of Man to Man, points out: "Seeing people with the same problem doing well years after diagnosis is very encouraging. It fulfills a real need. It gives men an extra push to go on living." Dr. Julia H. Rowland, a renowned expert in the field of psychooncology, claims that this kind of support can actually function as a vital element in healing:

> One of the most important "buffers" against the harm-
> ful effects of the stress of illness is the presence or avail-
> ability of people with whom the experience can be
> shared.... Research indicates that the presence of posi-
> tive social support not only diminishes the psychic dis-
> tress of cancer, but may be important in modulating
> survival as well.

Shop around among the available support groups to deter-mine the one that best suits you. You may even find that you and/or your partner prefer a more general (and, possibly, larger) cancer support group to a group that is focused specifically on prostate cancer.

Some prostate cancer support groups—for example, most Us Too groups—welcome both patients and caregivers to all regular meetings. Others, like most Man to Man groups, invite caregivers only once a quarter, on the theory that many men might be more willing to share their sexual, urinary, or psychological difficul-ties in a same-sex, all-patient environment than in a mixed one. A few groups (including some Man to Man groups) offer concurrent but separate meetings for patients and caregivers.

Neither you nor your partner should feel that you have to be a patient in crisis to be accepted in a support group or to derive benefit from it. Often men join a support group *while awaiting* the official diagnosis of prostate cancer, so that they'll have people around them who can help them deal with bad news. Frequently caregivers join or continue attending groups *after* their partner has died—not just to derive solace from others who are uniquely capable of appreciating their situation but also to share their own special knowledge and understanding with people in crisis.

Check with your doctor and local hospitals to find out what cancer and prostate-cancer support groups exist in your area. Here are some other leads:

◊ *Us Too*
Henry Porterfield
930 North York Road, Suite 50
Hinsdale, IL 60521-2993
800-808-7866

◊ In Canada contact: Norm Oman, Canadian coordinator of *Us Too*
53 Trafford Park
Winnipeg, Man. R2M 4Z7
204-257-6453 (fax)
204-257-6753 (phone)

◊ *American Foundation for Urologic Disease*
300 West Pratt Street, Suite #401
Baltimore, MD 21201
800-242-2383

◊ *Man to Man*
Contact your local American Cancer Society office, or call 800-ACS-2345

Information on Therapies and Health Care

The following organizations offer free or for-sale booklets, newsletters, or services of special interest to prostate cancer patients and their caregivers:

◊ *American Cancer Society* (all aspects of cancer)
1599 Clifton Road, NE
Atlanta, GA 30329
404-320-3333 (also check local listings; or call 800-ACS-2345 for local information)

Publications (free):

"Facts on Prostate Cancer"

"Listen with Your Heart"

"What Is Chemotherapy?"

"Radiation Therapy and You"

"For Men Only: Prostate Cancer"

◊ *National Cancer Institute* (all aspects of cancer)
Office of Cancer Communications
Building 31, Room 10A24
Bethesda, MD 20892
800-4-CANCER (800-422-6237)
services: Cancer Information Service (specific questions answered; English- and Spanish-speaking)
Physician Data Query (computerized database for questions relating to all types of cancer prevention, diagnosis, and treatment: available to doctors and patients)

Publications (free):

"Advanced Cancer: Living Each Day"

"Answers to Your Questions about Metastatic Cancer"

"Chemotherapy and You"

"Control of Cancer Pain Fact Sheet"

"Eating Hints: Recipes and Tips for Better Nutrition during Cancer Treatment"

"Questions and Answers about Pain Control"

"Radiation Therapy and You"

"Research Report: Cancer of the Prostate"

"Services Available for People with Cancer—National and Regional Organizations"

"Taking Time: Support for People with Cancer and the People Who Care about Them"

"What You Need to Know about Prostate Cancer"

'When Cancer Recurs: Meeting the Challenge Again"

◊ *Help for Incontinent People* (incontinence)
P.O. Box 8310
Spartanburg, SC 29305
803-579-7900

◊ *PAACT* (all prostate cancer treatments)
Lloyd Ney
P.O. Box 141695
1143 Parmelee NW
Grand Rapids, MI 49504
616-453-1477
quarterly newsletter (subscription): *Cancer Communication*

Recommended Reading

Borysenko, Joan. 1987. *Minding the Body, Mending the Mind.* Reading, MA: Addison-Wesley Publishing Co., Inc.

Broyard, Anatole. 1992. *Intoxicated by My Illness.* New York: Fawcett Columbine.

Dossey, Larry. 1991. *Meaning and Medicine.* New York: Bantam Books.

Fanning, Patrick. 1988. *Visualization for Change.* Oakland, CA: New Harbinger Publications, Inc.

Fiore, Neil A. 1984. *The Road Back to Health.* Berkeley, CA: Celestial Arts.

Gomella, Leonard G., and John J. Fried. 1993. *Recovering from Prostate Cancer.* New York: HarperCollins Publishers, Inc.

Haber, Sandra, ed. 1995. *Breast Cancer: A Psychological Treatment Manual.* New York: Springer Publishing Co., Inc.

Harpham, Wendy S. 1994. *After Cancer.* New York: W. W. Norton & Co., Inc.

Lerner, Michael. 1994. *Choices in Healing.* Cambridge, MA: The MIT Press.

LeShan, Lawrence. 1990. *Cancer as a Turning Point.* New York: Penguin USA.

Morganstern, Steven, and Allen Abrahams. 1993. *The Prostate Sourcebook.* Los Angeles: Lowell House.

Morra, Marion, and E. Potts. 1980. *Choices: Realistic Alternatives in Cancer Treatment.* New York: Avon Books.

Moyers, Bill. 1993. *Healing and the Mind.* New York: Doubleday.

Mullan, Fitzhugh, Barbara Hoffman, and the Editors of Consumer Reports Books. 1990. *An Almanac of Practical Resources for Cancer Survivors.* Mount Vernon, NY: Consumers Union.

Phillips, Robert H. 1994. *Coping with Prostate Cancer.* Garden City Park, NY: Avery Publishing Group, Inc.

Price, Reynolds. 1994. *A Whole New Life.* New York: Atheneum, Publishers.

Rosenblum, Daniel. 1993. *A Time to Hear, a Time to Help.* New York: The Free Press.

Simonton, O. Carl, and R. Henson. 1992. *The Healing Journey.* New York: Bantam Books.

Simonton, O. Carl, and S. Matthews-Simonton. 1980. *Getting Well Again.* New York: Bantam Books.

Vineyard, Sue. 1987. *How to Take Care of You.* Downers Grove, IL: Heritage Arts Publishing.

Index

E

H

I

O

P

R

S

W

X

Z

Barbara Rubin Wainrib, Ed.D., is a clinical psychologist in private practice in Montreal and adjunct professor at McGill University. She is the author of *Gender Issues Across the Life Cycle* and *Crisis Intervention and Trauma Response: Theory and Practice.*

Sandra Haber, Ph.D., is a psychologist in private practice in New York City. She is the editor of *Breast Cancer: A Psychological Treatment Manual.*

Drs. Wainrib and Haber are media consultants and lecture frequently to professional and lay audiences in the United States and Canada.

Jack Maguire is the author of twenty-four books, many in the areas of health, medicine, and psychology.

The foreword was contributed by **Michael Droller,** M.D., Mount Sinai Medical Center, New York, Medical Consultant.

Other books by Dr. Barbara Rubin Wainrib

Gender Issues Across the Life Cycle

Crisis Intervention and Trauma Response:
Theory and Practice

Edited by Dr. Sandra Haber

Breast Cancer: A Psychological Treatment Manual

More New Harbinger Titles

THE CHRONIC PAIN CONTROL WORKBOOK

A team of specialists in all areas of pain management detail the treatment strategies for managing and recovering from chronic pain.
Item PN2 Paperback $17.95

FIBROMYALGIA & CHRONIC MYOFASCIAL PAIN SYNDROME

This survival manual is the first comprehensive patient guide for managing these conditions. Readers learn how to identify trigger points, cope with chronic pain and sleep problems, and deal with the numbing effects of "fibrofog."   *Item FMS Paperback, $19.95*

OVERCOMING REPETITIVE MOTION INJURIES THE ROSSITER WAY

This system of easy-to-learn stretches has brought pain relief to thousands who suffer from carpal tunnel syndrome and other repetitive motion injuries and from everyday aches and pains.   *Item ROSS Paperback, $15.95*

PERIMENOPAUSE

Beginning with subtle changes in the mid-thirties and forties, perimenopause can encompass a bewildering array of symptoms. This self-care guide helps women assure health and vitality in the years ahead.
Item PERI Paperback, $16.95

TAKING CONTROL OF TMJ

Learn how to improve jaw functioning, relieve pain, eliminate harmful habits, and improve diet and exercise habits.   *Item TMJ Paperback $13.95*

Call **toll-free 1-800-748-6273** to order. Have your Visa or Mastercard number ready. Or send a check for the titles you want to New Harbinger Publications, 5674 Shattuck Avenue, Oakland, CA 94609. Include $3.80 for the first book and 75¢ for each additional book to cover shipping and handling. (California residents please include appropriate sales tax.) Allow four to six weeks for delivery.

Prices subject to change without notice.